A HISTORY OF THE QUEEN'S NURSING INSTITUTE

MONICA E. BALY

CROOM HELM
London & Sydney

© 1987 The Queen's Nursing Institute
Croom Helm Ltd, Provident House,
Burrell Row, Beckenham, Kent BR3 1AT
Croom Helm Australia, 44-50 Waterloo Road,
North Ryde, 2113, New South Wales

British Library Cataloguing in Publication Data
Baly, Monica E.
    A history of the Queen's Nursing Institute.
    1. Queen's Nursing Institute — History
    I. Title
    610.73′43′06041   RT98
    ISBN 0-7099-2107-1

Printed and bound in Great Britain by
Biddles Ltd, Guildford and King's Lynn

Contents

My view you know is that the ultimate destination of all nursing is the nursing of the sick in their own homes. . . . I look to the abolition of all hospitals and workhouse infirmaries. But it is no use to talk about the year 2,000.

Florence Nightingale to Mr Henry Bonham Carter, 4 June 1867

Plates

Foreword

This history of the Queen's Nursing Institute marks the centenary of its formal foundation with funds raised to celebrate another great anniversary, Queen Victoria's Golden Jubilee. The foundation was a crucial milestone in the development of a concept — the nursing of people, poor people, in their own homes and teaching them the rudiments of health care. This had been pioneered elsewhere, notably by my great-grandfather, the sixth William Rathbone, in Liverpool. He, with those great founding figures whose contributions you will find recorded here, set the standards and provided the impetus which have been maintained to this day.

The history of the Queen's Nursing Institute under its various names is a matter for pride, and over 50 years of working with and for the Institute have proved to me that its successes and contributions to the health of this country arise from using the past as a springboard for the future. As circumstances change, so must the course be changed and at each stage in its history the Institute has succeeded in so doing. But it can only continue to do so if it maintains its sense of vision (or perhaps mission would be a better word) as to how community nursing, district nursing, can best be made to be a major contributor to the health and thus the quality of life at every level of society. This we can do through nurse training; through nurse education; as a focus for our district and community nurses; as a source of pride.

This history shows what has been achieved and these achievements provide the launching pad for the next hundred years. The Institute must not, and I am sure will not, fail to continue to find the new ways forward.

William Rathbone

Acknowledgements

I accepted the task of writing this book at the request of the Council of the Queen's Nursing Institute who placed their archival material at my disposal. I am grateful to the Council and the staff at the Institute who have given me every assistance, and my particular thanks are due to Mr Philip Starr, the Chief Administrator, who has acted as a guide and counsellor throughout. I am also grateful to Mrs Martin Acland, the Chairman of the Institute for her advice and criticism and to members of the Council who read the script and made suggestions. I am particularly grateful to Dr Charlotte Kratz for her advice and to Mrs Dorothy Jones who read the later chapters with me and corrected my errors.

The records of the Institute are like their empire, far flung. There is a wealth of material about early district nursing in the British Library and my thanks go to the trustees, particularly in relation to the access to the Nightingale/Rathbone papers. I am also grateful to the librarians of the Greater London Record Office where I had access to the Bonham Carter papers and much of Miss Nightingale's and Miss Lee's correspondence on district nursing. The Queen's Institute inspector's reports, where they are preserved, are lodged with the Public Record Office at Kew; these often provide a vivid picture of the life of a Queen's nurse in an earlier period, and I acknowledge the help given by the librarians in working the system. The Picton Library in Liverpool was most helpful in finding boxes of material relating to the Liverpool District Nursing Association and the early Queen's nurses in Liverpool. My thanks are also due to the library of the Royal College of Nursing and to its History Room and its treasures of early nursing books and journals and to Miss Alison Bramley who helped with access to the records of the Public Health Section. Before I began I was helped by advice from Dr Bynum of the Wellcome Institute for the History of Medicine, and from Lesley Hall who catalogued the archives at the Queen's Nursing Institute.

On reading the material in the Institute I found that Miss Merry and Miss Crothers had previously sorted and prepared early material in a 'precious letters' file when they acted as assistants to Mrs Mary Stocks in 1957; this proved a valuable starting point and I only hope what I have produced has been worthy of their research. My thanks are also due to Dr Donaldson who made available to me material from her own research on district nursing in Ireland. I am also grateful to the help given by Miss Barbara Robottom, the Professional Nursing Officer at the English National Board, on the more recent events.

But my greatest thanks go to the Queen's nurses themselves. I feel this history is like Elgar's Enigma Variations, 'my friends pictured within'. Apart from the Queen's nurses who have sent me their recollections, this book is a tribute to the many Queen's nurses I knew when I was an Area Organiser for the Royal College of Nursing in the 1950s and 1960s who often gave me hospitality. Not only did I see the work of the nurses first hand in those days, but often, staying with them, I heard the recollections of the Queen's in the 1930s. In this respect I would like to pay particular tribute to the late Miss Ann White MBE and Miss Dora Williams OBE, from whom I learned much. I also record with thanks the late Miss Edith Bussby who was an officer at the Institute until she retired in 1972, who discussed with me 'the world we have lost' and whose title we agreed together, and who recalled life as a district nurse before the war.

Preface

It is a hundred years since the Queen's Nursing Institute was founded as Queen Victoria's Jubilee Institute for Nurses. The most remarkable achievement of the Queen's Institute is its longevity. Most Victorian charities for the poor sick have disappeared or suffered a sea change into something, if not rich, often strange. A hundred years on, the Queen's Institute continues to honour its Charter by providing training and educational opportunities for district nurses. That it is now further education is a measure of how well the Institute fulfilled its primary task when, after a long struggle, the district nurse training which it had pioneered was recognised as a statutory requirement.

The fact that the Institute, with a comparatively small income, managed to survive in a rapidly changing world is largely due to the ingenuity of its Council in adapting to social change and sometimes tempering the shorn lamb to the wind and somehow surviving the various financial crises. It is, however, also due to the fact that the Queen's Nurses themselves were flexible and adaptable; they took on duties and shed them, as advances in medicine and the new needs of the population demanded. This history has endeavoured to trace these two strands.

First, the philosophy and policies of the Institute, at each point in history, must be seen in the light of the politics and social change taking place around it. Whether it was the economic depression at the end of the nineteenth century, the Liberal reforms of the early part of this century and the first stirrings of state intervention in medicine, interwar unemployment, the coming of the National Health Service and finally new concepts of nursing education, the Institute has to adapt its policy.

Founded to serve the poor sick, 'the poorest of the Queen's subjects', and supported by voluntary donations, nevertheless, the Institute wished to establish a universal nursing service that would provide a standard of excellence and act as a grain of mustard seed. This was its dilemma — how to accomplish both aims. The Council believed strongly in the voluntary ideal, but with each step towards state medicine they cleverly managed to sell at least some of their services to public authorities. Sometimes they were poorly paid for their efforts, but that they managed to do so and survive as a training body until well into the NHS says much for the persuasive powers of the Council, but also much for the regard in which the Queen's nurses were held by the public. The new broom of state medicine did not dare disregard the public affection for Queen's nurses.

It is important to see the history of the Queen's Institute within the context of the contemporary social ethos. We must read history in the situation in which it occurred and not in the light of our own preoccupations. Mr Rathbone, Miss Nightingale and Miss Lees were as avant garde in their prescription for health care in their day as anything the health service has produced. Miss Loane and her colleagues, imbued with the ideas of the Eugenics Movement and uplifting the worthy poor through education, were as revolutionary in 1908 as were Professor Black's 'Inequalities of Health Care' report in 1981.

It is fitting that the hundred years of the Queen's Institute should end with the training that they founded being mandatory and with future hopes that a Neighbourhood Nursing Service will be introduced in which some of the divisions between health workers in the community will eventually be overcome. At the same time it is appropriate that the hundred years of health mission should coincide with the World Health Declaration at Alma Ata with its aim of health for all by AD 2000, an aim which the founders of the Institute would have approved, but for which time is running out.

Monica E. Baly

1

Nursing the Sick Poor at Home Before 1887

People have always cared for the sick at home. Nor is compassion for the sick a Christian prerogative. Thucydides, writing about the terrible plague that visited Athens in 429 BC says that people visited the sick to give them attention and in so doing lost their lives; this was particularly true of those 'who made it a point of honour to act properly'.[1] Caring for the sick was a Pauline exhortation, and those early deaconesses like Phoebe who did so received the praise that St Paul rarely bestowed on women. The tradition was carried on by the medieval Church and it is significant that the monasteries, already in decline in the fourteenth century, never recovered from the effects of the plague of 1348 and the following years on their personnel. Whatever the failings of the Church Militant, it apparently did its duty to its sick flock both in hospices and in their own homes.

EARLY ATTEMPTS

One of the first attempts to train women for nursing the sick at home came during the Catholic reformation in France and was made by St Vincent de Paul. First he appealed to the instincts of good women to form Associations of Charities and visit the sick at home for whom he supplied nursing rules. Later, in 1633, he started his great work in Paris where, under the direction of Mlle Le Gras, he recruited suitable country girls as nurses who were taken into a nurses' home and given a training in home nursing including such skills as 'using a lancet, the tourniquet and applying poultices'.[2] These *soeurs de charité*, like others in orders set up during the Counter Reformation, nursed both in institutions and the poor in their own homes. The Sisters of Mercy are important because in the nineteenth century Miss

1

Nightingale and other would-be nurse reformers went to Paris to study their methods, and, in the Crimean war, William Howard Russell, the correspondent of *The Times*, held them up as a shining example and a shame to England who lacked such a nursing force. In the event, the motley band under Miss Nightingale not only emulated the French, but in matters of hygiene and organisation surpassed them.

Protestant England, however, was not entirely un-nursed. Whilst medicine was unscientific and life expectancy about 30 years, there was little call for organised nursing, but for the sick poor who were unsupported by family or neighbours there were those twin pillars of English social policy: the Poor Law and charities. Until the Amendment Act of 1834 most Poor Law relief was given as 'outdoor'. Every parish was a petty kingdom and a law unto itself, but it is now generally accepted that in the eighteenth and early nineteenth century the Guardians and Overseers often dealt with the sick in a humane way. Many parishes employed doctors and nurses who visited the sick at home. In the Bath records we read of a Nurse Philpot dispensing senna and salts and being allowed money for brimstone and treacle and for 'staying with a woman with smallpox'.[3] In a neighbouring parish the nurses did the vaccinations and no one asked 'what is the proper task of the nurse?' Parish nurses employed by the Guardians were giving service until well into the twentieth century. In 1870 the Liverpool Ladies' Committee 'agreed to take fever patients and the services of the Parish nurse unaccompanied by relief from the Parish . . . '.[4] At a conference of Queen's nurses in 1912 it was claimed, with pride, that in some places in London Queen's nurses 'had almost taken over from parish nurses'. Not all parish nursing was bad. Reformers tend to overstate their case.

THE EARLY NINETEENTH CENTURY

Apart from the Guardians, in the early nineteenth century there were a growing number of charities; this was partly due to the religious zeal of Methodism and the new Dissent, partly to the growing affluence of the middle classes, but largely to the fear of riot and rebellion engendered by the French revolution. Visiting societies sprang up and gave tickets to beggars to get them off the streets and invited them to an office where gentlemen of the committee took a case history and if necessary visited the 'deserving' in their homes; these were given practical help and if sick, as many were, neighbours were dragooned or a nurse hired, and the Society supervised.[5] The

Ladies' Committee visited with advice on child care, layettes and tracts about vaccination; they were in fact early health visitors.

With the publication of Edwin Chadwick's *Report on the Sanitary Conditions of the Labouring Population of Great Britain* in 1842, and the reports of doctors like Arnott, Kay and Southwood Smith, the reading public began to see the connection between insanitary conditions, disease and the burden on the poor-rate. Not only was there a connection between disease, dirt and pauperism, there was also a link between poor housing and crime and this gave a new impetus to Health of Towns Associations and visiting societies. Better housing and better health, it was argued, would raise the moral standard of the lower classes. In Oxford during the cholera outbreak of 1854 the Guardians decided that medical attendance should be provided for the houses of the poor:

> A list was kept of all respectable women who were willing to nurse in Cholera houses. The names have been furnished mainly through the knowledge of the local clergy. . . . When a new case was announced in the house of any poor person a messenger proceeded from the Post Office to the house of a nurse 'returned home' and sent her to where her help was required. . . . and lastly because most important, a lady visited every house to instruct the nurses to comfort the sick, to cheer the disconsolate and where the need was, herself to supply a sudden emergency or relieve the wearied attendant.[6]

Here, as with the *soeurs de charité* and the visiting societies, a lady supervised the nurse, a tradition that the Liverpool Ladies' Committee were to take over.

The urbanisation fostered by the industrial revolution and the growing misery of the poor in the midst of increasing affluence acted as a spur to conscience. Although many denominations set up charities for the poor, two groups are particularly associated with home nursing; the Quakers and the Anglican Oxford Movement. Mrs Elizabeth Fry met Paster Fliedner, the founder of the German Deaconess system, when he was in England in 1822 and she herself visited Kaiserswerths on the Rhine, that Mecca of nursing reformers, and returned determined to set up a similar system in England. In the event Mrs Fry's work on penal reform prevented her from playing an active part in the work, but with the help of her sister, Mrs Gurney, and her daughters, in 1840 she started the Society of Protestant Sisters of Charity, which at the suggestion of the Dowager Queen Adelaide, the patron, was eventually called the Institute of Nursing Sisters. The committee was distinguished and Mrs Fry was received by the young Queen Victoria, possibly the Queen's first intimation of the growing need for home nursing among her poorer subjects.

The first minutes of the Institute record that 'many eligible persons offered themselves', and there is no doubt but that the ladies' committee were rigorous in scrutinising testimonials so that only worthy candidates were accepted. The successful were sent to Guy's Hospital or the London for some training where no doubt they learnt something of the little that medical science had to teach in 1841. The sisters were issued with a uniform, and it is perhaps not surprising that in April 1841 the committee had to deal with an item on the agenda that read 'objections having been reported of some of the elected sisters relative to the dress'.[7] In history things happen earlier than is supposed.

The sisters were given free board, lodging and clothing and were paid a small stipend; they lived in an institution and were supervised by a paid superintendent, which is much as the arrangement was for the first Nightingale nurses some 20 years later. However, the sisters had to earn their keep and they were sent to paid employment in private families and this is where the scheme fell down. When they were not so employed the sisters' 'leisure time is devoted to the nursing of the sick in the densely peopled and wretched districts that immediately surround their home'.[8]

How much time was given to the nursing of the poor is doubtful, but correspondence between Mrs Gurney and a Dr West gives some idea of what was expected of the sisters:

> She would be required to learn by daily enquiry whether any instructions had been left for her at the dispensary . . . she would then visit any poor whose names had been entered in the book and if ordered would do any of those little duties that a nurse may be required to perform, as making and applying poultices, applying leeches etc. . . . She should endeavour to teach the poor how they might themselves perform any of the duties she has to execute. For instance she might teach them how to stop bleeding from leech bites, how to dress a blister, how to make poultices etc. She would also be skilled in cheap cookery for the sick. Her duties should be rather those of an instructress.[9]

Sentiments with which neither Miss Nightingale nor Miss Lees would later quarrel.

The importance of the Institute was the stress that it laid on the sisters being 'worthy' with high ethical standards, but in fact it failed to make much impact because the numbers were few, it was confused in its aims and the training was too brief. There was the continuing debate as to whether the sisters should give their services for money 'to persons of comparative refinement but who are in circumstances of great limitation', and thus pay their way, or gratuitously to the 'necessitous poor', a debate that did not end with Mrs Fry's deaconesses. It seems likely from the minutes that the sisters preferred 'persons of comparative refinement'.

In 1833 John Keble preached his famous sermon in Oxford on 'national apostasy' and set in train a series of pamphlets called 'Tracts for our Times', from which was derived the name Tractarian. The Oxford Movement, as it was called, sought to revive the ideals of the Anglican Church and place greater relative importance on good works as against the predestination of the Calvinists. This emphasis on good works led to the formation of 'orders', some of which were devoted to nursing. One such group was run by Miss Sellon and the Bishop of Exeter who nursed the cholera patients in Devonport in the 1850s; another was the Reverend Pusey's group, the Park Village Community, who nursed around Regent's Park.

But perhaps the best known was the order of St John the Evangelist, based on the parish of St John in St Pancras and founded by the Bishop of London assisted by Dr Todd and Dr William Bowman, Miss Nightingale's 'dear friend' and correspondent of many years. This order was divided into three: probationers who did two years' training in hospitals; nurses who 'nursed' and were paid a wage; and sisters who instructed. St John's and similar institutions provided 'trained nurses' to hospitals for a fixed sum; they also provided nurses for home nursing. Miss Mary Jones, Miss Nightingale's 'dearest friend', whose correspondence with her helps to fill some of the lacunae about the problems of the Nightingale School, became the Superintendent in 1854 supplying six nurses for Scutari and in 1856 took over the nursing at King's College Hospital and later at Charing Cross. These nursing orders are important because it was imagined — and feared — that Miss Nightingale would use the Nightingale Fund to found such an order. However, Miss Nightingale had learnt her lesson with the 'Lady Ecclesiastics' in the Crimea and was insistent that the Nightingale School, when it did come, should be non-sectarian, an article of faith that was to be handed on to district nursing.

In the mid-nineteenth century, therefore, there were a number of nursing organisations providing care in hospitals and to the sick at home. Of course they did not meet the rising demand, but that was not a phenomenon peculiar to the nineteenth century. District nursing did not begin *de novo* in 1860, 1874 or even in 1887. It is a seamless cloth with a few women responding to the needs of each age in light of the medical and sanitary theories of the time.

1850 TO 1887

In 1856 when Miss Nightingale returned from the Crimea her first thought was not to reform nursing but the army medical service, and if necessary the army itself. She regarded the Nightingale Fund, subscribed to help her train nurses and hospital attendants, as a millstone because she had no time, and no clear plan, as to how such a training could be carried out or by whom.[10] After two years of delay and toying with the idea of latching the Fund to St John's, the Fund Council agreed to accept the offer of St Thomas's as a 'humble beginning' with fifteen probationers under the supervision of Mrs Wardroper, the matron of St Thomas's, who under the terms of the agreement was also to be head of the training school.

In 1860, before the training was under way, Miss Nightingale received a letter, and later a visit, from a Mr William Rathbone who was the eldest son of a dynasty of Liverpool merchants and the sixth William Rathbone in succession to be a senior partner in the family firm. Born in 1819, a year before Miss Nightingale, he had inherited a family tradition of philanthropy and liberalism; his family had originally been Quakers and had taken a leading part in the campaign for Catholic emancipation. Now he was a Unitarian and an honorary visitor to the District Provident Society in one of the poorest districts of Liverpool. His attitude and credentials appealed to Miss Nightingale and there was a rapport between them that was to last for over 40 years. Mr Rathbone was later to write 'in matters of nursing Miss Nightingale is my Pope'.

One reason for the letter was that during 1859 Mr Rathbone's wife had been nursed in her last illness by a Mrs Mary Robinson, who possibly trained with St John's and who had proved such a comfort to the patient and the family that it occurred to Mr Rathbone 'to engage Mrs Robinson to go into the poorest districts of Liverpool and try, in nursing the poor, to relieve suffering and teach them the rules of health and comfort.[11] After a month or so Mrs Robinson returned crying, saying that she could no longer bear the misery she saw, but Mr Rathbone persuaded her to continue and she eventually became enthusiastic and stayed for another four years nursing the poor. Mr Rathbone was encouraged and determined to pursue the experiment, but the problem was where to find suitable nurses, and he sought advice from Miss Nightingale, nationally famous and about to start the Nightingale School. Originally there was correspondence with Arthur Clough, the secretary of the Nightingale Fund, who answered for Miss Nightingale, and who advised that Liverpool should train their own nurses, and the Liverpool Committee should build a Nurses' Home; Sir Joshua Jebb, the then chairman of the Nightingale Fund, was asked to give help with the construction. In 1860 Mr Rathbone and the committee formulated plans which he set out in a long letter to Miss Nightingale.

> We think of having a superior nurse in the central ward of each set of wards and in that ward a probationer. After having been four months in that ward she will move to one of the other two wards, then four months night nursing will make up her year. This whole time she will be under the same training sister. I attach as much importance to missionary nursing as hospital. . . . As we find nurses for missionary work we shall offer them to ministers of religion and other efficient kind people in different parts of the town who will form local committees and raise amongst themselves funds for medical comforts and find proper superintendence.[12]

Miss Nightingale was critical of the training plan, especially the idea of nurses training under the same sister, though interestingly enough she does not question the sister's ability to give instruction. On 20 June she sent a long letter starting: 'I have thought a good deal over the Liverpool plans as I would if I were going to be matron myself.' She then goes on to set forth her views as she held them in 1860 about the importance of female staff living in the hospital and in rooms off wards.

> This facilitates the manager's task, prevents gossip and promotes the efficiency of the nurses. . . . A common day room is undesirable. It encourages dawdling and gossiping. Her time ought to be fully occupied by her ward work, her necessary sleep and exercise and what making and mending she has to do for herself. . . .[13]

There is nothing in this long letter about instruction for nurses, and no advice about training district nurses. At this stage Miss

Nightingale was aiming at working-class girls and the first objective was to keep them fully occupied, away from gossip or the corrupting influences of corridors or airing courts. The journey to the Nurses' Home should be as infrequent and as exposed as possible. Nurses should be supervised at all times.

Although Mr Rathbone was grateful for the advice he received, it is doubtful whether it was particularly helpful to his needs, and it was Mary Jones of King's College Hospital who gave the most practical advice. Mr Rathbone, now married again to a wife who shared his philanthropic ideals, pursued his plans. The training school and the Nurses' Home were financed by Mr Rathbone himself and when the Home was extended later the cost was defrayed by the Rathbone family firm. He, and the Central Relief Committee of Liverpool with whom he worked in close cooperation, saw his missionary scheme as not only relieving sickness but as being morally uplifting.

> after the nurse had shown what might be done to restore order the husbands who were well meaning, industrious men took heart again and left off drinking and were saved together with their families from the utter state of degradation and wretchedness into which they were sinking when the nurse came to the rescue.[14]

This was a sentiment with which Miss Nightingale would have agreed as she was fond of saying that the district nurse 'may be the forerunners in teaching the disorderly how to use imperfect dwellings, teaching without seeming to teach'.[15]

The nurse as a moral agent and as a means of combating pauperism was a strong argument put forward by nineteenth-century reformers to support their case that nurses needed to be worthy, respectable, morally earnest and trained. Nurses were heeded, so the argument ran, not because they were clever, but because they were good women and disciplined.

In 1861 it was difficult to find worthy women for such a task in Liverpool or elsewhere. Mr Rathbone found two ladies, Elizabeth and Mary Merryweather, and sent them to St Thomas's to observe the Nightingale School. They did not sign the regulations, and it is doubtful what they observed as the thirteen probationers had by then moved to the Surrey Gardens and were working under poor and difficult conditions with little supervision. Four Nightingale nurses returned with the Misses Merryweather to Liverpool; one soon died of typhus and the other three were of doubtful value. Miss Merryweather had to recruit and train at Liverpool with little or no experience; later Miss Nightingale said of Elizabeth 'does she know *anything* about nursing?' But within the light of the times, the scant advice given, the scheme set up by Mr and Mrs Rathbone for organising district nursing in Liverpool becomes understandable.

The city was divided into numbered districts based on the parishes of Liverpool and ministers of religion were asked to cooperate though the work was to be strictly non-sectarian, a principle that was to raise some difficulties with the ministers of religion later. Each district had a committee and was in the charge of a lady superintendent. The supervision of nurses by ladies was not unique: Mrs Fry's committee did it, the ladies of Oxford did it and Miss Nightingale wrote apropos Liverpool:

> I do not mean these efforts are new and original but I mean it is most satisfactory to find the Lady Superintendent and nurse exercising certain powers and influences in Sanitary matters such as obtaining the cleansing and limewashing of unhealthy houses and places.[16]

Lady superintendents there could be, and if ladies interested themselves in drains so much the better.

It is clear from the Liverpool Ladies' Committee minute book that the poverty in Liverpool in the 1860s was so great and the unemployment so high that the first problem was not nursing but the sheer relief of hunger and the provision of shelter, and most of the entries are about the giving of relief rather than nursing cases. The situation is set out by Charles Langton, Mr Rathbone's collaborator, in a long letter to Miss Nightingale in 1869.

> The work lies with the poor and destitute in courts and cellars, many families in one house in dirt and degradation. [In the] Districts we have half-trained nurses, others worked by women partly trained, or by reason of long experience qualified for dealing with those for whom they labour. Under the Superintendent there is a Lady Inspector who goes and enquires for herself into the general conduct and efficiency of the nurse. Some Lady Superintendents prefer all untrained nurses, others cannot afford the expense. . . .[17]

Miss Nightingale's reply is not preserved, but later she was critical of the nursing in Liverpool. It seems obvious that nine years after the scheme had begun only half the districts had 'trained' nurses in

Liverpool and that not much importance was attached to employing them. The Royal Liverpool Infirmary was supplying not only nurses for the district but also for private families and for the hospital itself, and, as at St Thomas's, the wastage and turnover was high. In the circumstances the committee was probably right; the diseases of the poor living in cellars and airless courts were due to malnutrition, damp and contaminated water. What was needed was not nursing but employment at reasonable wages, better housing and main drainage.

Mr Rathbone's concept of district nursing spread to other towns. In 1867 Manchester sent to King's College and St Thomas's for nurses, and as in Liverpool nurses were engaged for district work, the hospital and private cases. On the district the nurses were supervised by the lady superintendent who reported that the district nurse was good with: 'trivial complaints that could develop, chronic illness unsuitable for hospital such as the various forms of malignant tumour popularly designated by the term 'cancer' (sic) and relapses of consumptive patients . . .'.[18] By the end of the 1860s there were a number of district nursing associations more or less on the Liverpool pattern with hospital-trained nurses and untrained nurses supervised by ladies.

The importance of the Liverpool experiment was that it inaugurated the idea that a district nurse should be a trained hospital nurse, preferably trained under the Nightingale reformed system. Liverpool introduced the idea of dividing a city or town into 'districts' each being organised by a lay committee with a lady superintendent to supervise the nurse. The Liverpool system was advocated in the 1860s and often copied, particularly in the north. When later Miss Lees, and then the Queen's Institute, introduced the idea of trained, educated nurse superintendents, with the nurses accountable to a nurse and not to a lady superintendent, this led to schism and was one reason why some associations did not affiliate with the Queen's Institute.

Back in London a Mrs Ranyard started a new venture in home nursing from a different perspective. An ardent supporter of the British and Foreign Bible Society, Mrs Ranyard was convinced that salvation could be brought to the nefarious area around Seven Dials if the inhabitants could be supplied with bibles. To this end she recruited missionary workers to sell bibles on the hire purchase system, and by 1864 there were 200 bible women working for the mission. Then, in 1868, it was decided that a small group of working class trained bible women should undertake the care of the sick in their districts, and for this purpose they were sent to Guy's Hospital for a three-month training which was later extended to a longer period. The bible nurse returned to her district under the supervision of the lady superintendent who endeavoured to collect funds and pennies from grateful patients to pay for the services of the nurses. The mission continued with considerable success and by the time Miss Lees did her survey in 1874, with the exception of the East London Nursing Society, it was the only organised body of trained nurses working exclusively in the homes of the poor in London.

In 1868 Mr Rathbone was elected as a Liberal MP for a division in Liverpool and now spent part of the year in London where he was in greater contact with Miss Nightingale. They corresponded regularly about district nursing and as early as 1867 Miss Nightingale was writing:

> I rejoice that your District Nursing is likely to be imitated in the East of London, you know I shall never think that we have done anything in London until we have nursed not only all the hospitals and all the workhouses, but have divided London into convenient districts for nursing the sick.[19]

In 1874 Sir Edward Lechmere of the English Branch of the Order of St John of Jerusalem proposed that a system of district nursing be inaugurated in London and that the Duke of Westminster be approached to help. Mr Rathbone and Miss Nightingale were obviously asked for advice and it is clear from the almost daily correspondence between them that Miss Nightingale made the pellets and Mr Rathbone fired the shots. The first resolution framed by Miss Nightingale was to persuade the committee to do a survey on the nursing needs of London and to take time to do it. Secondly, they agreed that the only person to conduct the survey was a Miss Florence Lees who seems to have converted Mr Rathbone to a new vision of district nursing, for he writes:

> I think there is a good chance of getting two good things tried. . . . Lady nurses for the poor — Miss Lees' ideal, and self-supporting sick nursing among the workmen. Bonham Carter and Mrs Senior are very anxious for the latter.[20]

Mr Rathbone sent a blow-by-blow account of the difficult committee meetings to Miss Nightingale in which he complains of fashionable ladies and fashionable doctors on the committee who would be of no assistance, but he assures her that the real work will be done by a subcommittee which will consist of the nominees he and she have

11

chosen together. *Plus ça change — plus c'est la même chose.* These included Henry Bonham Carter, the secretary of the Nightingale Fund and Miss Nightingale's cousin, who was to work for the cause of district nursing for the rest of his long life. Thus packed, the sub-committee agreed to the need for a survey and that Miss Florence Lees should be appointed to do it.

Florence Lees

Born in 1841 in comfortable circumstances at St Leonards where in her youth she accompanied her mother visiting the sick poor in the neighbourhood, Florence Lees decided that she wanted to nurse. In 1866 she went to St Thomas's, not as a probationer but to observe for four months because her mother would not let her be exposed to the rough and tumble of the nurse's life in the early Nightingale School. Mrs Wardroper, the matron of St Thomas's, did not like Miss Lees and wrote cryptically in the report book 'well educated, fair surgical nurse, did little training, did not comply with the regulations' the latter being a heinous crime in the eyes of Mrs Wardroper.

Florence Lees is interesting because she is an example of how well-educated, reasonably affluent young women like Agnes Jones, Jane Shaw Stewart and others could go around Europe visiting hospitals, with the inevitable spell at Kaiserswerth, and study nursing, with some paying for private tuition from surgeons, and return home equipped to be superintendents. In 1870 Miss Lees was nursing in France but at the advent of the Franco-Prussian war she was persuaded by the Crown Princess Frederick, the eldest daughter of Queen Victoria, to organise nursing in a military hospital in Prussia. Florence Lees was obviously liked and admired by the Crown Princess who continued to correspond with her and who, in later years, became a god-mother to her eldest son. This royal connection stood her in good stead when she returned home and later when she was appointed a member of the Council of the Queen Victoria's Jubilee Institute.

Having studied nursing in both Canada and in the United States, she returned to England to be persuaded by Miss Nightingale and the Crown Princess to 'harness her great cleverness' to some positive job, and although she wanted to go off on further study Mr Rathbone persuaded her to undertake the survey. The first question to be answered was: is there a need for a district nursing service in London? Miss Lees' report though probably tendentious and at times intolerant gives a splendid and detailed picture of the nursing scene in London in 1874, both in the major hospitals and in the districts.[21] Miss Lees visited all the training schools and set out a report rather like that prepared by a General Nursing Council inspector some 50 years later. The weighty appendices include a survey of the 22 nursing organisations providing district nursing in London, but of these the report says 'only one-third can be said to be trained at all'.

A main theme running through the report is the need to provide careers for educated women, and nursing, properly organised, offered this opportunity. District nursing should be undertaken, and supervised, by educated ladies who had been trained as nurses and not supervised by the laity who did not understand nursing and did not know how to use nurses. What is interesting about the report is that it is critical of all nurse training at that time, including that at St Thomas's: 'Even the improved training given at the Nightingale School does not supply the comprehensive education and training that should elevate nursing to the rank of the scientific art for educated women', and Miss Lees proceeds to argue for a two-tier system:

> Whether it would be possible to institute a higher grade of nurse, a superior education and such a system of training as would make nursing a profession in which a lady would not feel she was sacrificing herself, but on the contrary would feel that she was raising herself by entering a profession at once noble and honorable.[22]

This proposition, however, did not endear Miss Lees to Miss Nightingale who was of the firm opinion that the 'lady should be educated with her cook' and the one portal of entry that the nursing profession was to cling to until the Second World War. Nor did it necessarily please Mr Rathbone with his committees of ladies in Liverpool who wrote that he 'did not understand Miss Lees' views'. There is no doubt but that some of the disputatious episodes between Miss Lees and her committee, and indeed with Miss Nightingale, were due to her advanced ideas on nurse education and her insistence on recruiting 'ladies'. However, in spite of the fact that Miss Lees, in her report, was severe about Liverpool and had written 'there was no nursing going on there', Mr Rathbone accepted that in Liverpool they were behind the times and came round to the view that 'we need superior, educated, trained superintendents'.[23]

The new association took the cumbersome title of The Metropolitan and National Nursing Association, and Miss Nightingale espoused the cause heartily by writing a letter to *The Times* appealing for funds in which she shows herself converted to Miss Lees' view of district nursing:

A district nurse must first nurse. She must be of a yet higher class and of a yet fuller training than a hospital nurse, because she has no hospital appliances at hand at all; and because she has to take notes of the case for the doctor, who has no one but her to report to him. She is his staff of clinical clerks, dressers and nurses.[24]

Miss Lees was duly appointed Superintendent General of the new association and the Nightingale Fund not only promised donations but also offered to train 'special probationers' at the Nightingale School for district work; 'specials' were candidates judged to be fitted for superintendence; there was therefore a strong link with the Nightingale School. In 1877 Mr Rathbone became a trustee of the Nightingale Fund as did the Duke of Westminster, and of course, Henry Bonham Carter, the secretary of the Fund, helped to ensure that the association started on a firm foundation. As the Metropolitan and National was to become the working model for the Queen Victoria's Jubilee Institute this link is important, for it ensured that the training both in the hospital and on the district was on Nightingale lines with an emphasis on discipline — both on duty and off — and it accounts for the high proportion of Nightingale nurses among the early district nurses.

The Central Home of the Association was at 23 Bloomsbury Square, which provided the office for the Superintendent and comfortable accommodation for five district nurse probationers who did a special training. Letters from St Thomas's nurses who joined the staff suggest that the atmosphere was happier and freer than at St Thomas's, but they leave a vivid picture of the dire squalor of the district near the Home in the late 1870s. But all was not well. Miss Lees did not work in harmony with her committee, and time and again Miss Nightingale and Mr Bonham Carter had to intervene. There was trouble at the subsidiary home at Holloway where the ladies objected to the time they had to set out in the morning and where threats of mass resignations and a strike were only narrowly averted. At one stage Miss Nightingale wrote:

She [Miss Lees] has been treating us scurvily. . . . She has been doing this for 7 years, a mixture of flattering and trust most nauseous . . . but for the life of me I know no one that could start district nurses on their duties but Miss Lees.[25]

It is difficult to tell the truth from the conflicting evidence. Miss Lees' concept of the educated lady nurse went against the grain of some of her committee who tended to be chauvinistic men, and, reading between the lines, one gets the impression that Miss Lees did not always press her point tactfully. On the other hand Miss Nightingale was not always wise in *her* judgement and she tended to exaggerate, and, in spite of the fulsome letters of later years, she was not always in harmony with Mr Rathbone of whom at one stage she said: 'Mistakes the functions of such a society [the Metropolitan and National] for those of a London Board School or the Charity Organisation Society'.[26] Meanwhile, Mr Bonham Carter poured oil on the troubled waters around the ladies of Holloway. It was not only Miss Lees who was difficult.

In 1878, Miss Lees, aged 37 years, became engaged to and married the Reverend Dacre Craven, the Rector of St George the Martyr, who lived round the corner in Great Ormond Street, was a great supporter of the work and shared her views. The Reverend Dacre Craven became secretary to the Central Home. He was handsome and well liked by the committee and in 1889 he was invited to join the Nightingale Fund Council which he served faithfully until 1918; he was also a prime mover in the early work of the Queen Victoria's Jubilee Institute bringing to it, with his wife, the experience and ideals of the Metropolitan and National Nursing Association. According to memoirs it was a happy marriage; Mrs Dacre Craven was a good housekeeper, hostess and mother and she was devoted to her husband, and for some years she continued her superintendence of the Home in Bloomsbury on an unpaid basis. In 1899 Mrs Craven published *A Guide to District Nurses and Home Nursing* which was duly proof-read by Miss Nightingale who subsequently held up Mrs Craven as a paragon as far as district nursing was concerned. The *Guide* sets out the thesis that district nurses need to be of a superior education and they need special training to equip them to work in the homes of the poor. But superior education does not mean condescension: 'The district nurses must be content to be the servant of the poor sick and the teacher by turns. Wherever she enters order and cleanliness must enter with her'; and there follows much practical advice about nursing and nursing ethics and the improvisation of equipment with which succeeding generations of district nurses have had no wish to quarrel.

Florence Lees must be seen as the true originator, not of district nursing, but of professional district nursing with a special and higher training where the nurse was accountable, not to a lady superintendent, but to a highly trained nurse. To this concept she converted both Miss Nightingale and Mr Rathbone, and it says much for Mr

Rathbone's flexibility that he was so converted. It is fortunate that the Metropolitan and National Nursing Association was formed at a time when the idea of the trained nurse was taking root, and when, after a doubtful start, there were a few educated women with leadership ability taking up nursing and ready to pioneer new ventures. It is also fortunate that the Association coincided with the greater acceptance of scientific medicine, Listerian surgery, asepsis and the germ theory, and, above all, with new ideas about the emancipation of educated women into paid occupations. The ethos of district nurses going out from their comfortable home in Bloomsbury in their smart uniforms, arguing with their superintendent about their starting time was very different from that of Mrs Fry's respectable women, or indeed the nurses of Liverpool in the 1860s who were mainly concerned with welfare. Not only had there been 20 years of nurse training, however inefficient and unscientific Miss Lees and other critics deemed it, women were now seeking worthwhile careers and promotion. In Miss Nightingale's words nursing had become fashionable.

This, then, was the new concept of district nursing when Queen Victoria celebrated her Golden Jubilee in 1887.

NOTES

1. Thucydides, (trans. R. Warner), *The Peloponnesian War*, Penguin Classics, 1954, p.126.

2. Baly, M.E. *Nursing and Social Change*, Heinemann, London, 2nd Edn, 1982, p. 44.

3. Overseers Account Books St Peter and St Paul (Bath) Poor Relief Book 1800–11. County Record Department, Taunton.

4. Ladies Committee Minute Book (Liverpool) October 1870.

5. Turner, P. Vere. *History of the Monmouth St Society 1805–1905*, Godwin, Bath 1905.

6. Acland, Sir W. *Memoirs of the Cholera Epidemic at Oxford in 1854*, Churchill, London, 1856, pp. 98–9.

7. Institute of Nursing Sisters, Raven Row, Whitechapel, Minute Book April 1841.

8. *A History of the Nursing Sister's Institute*, Shearn Bros. London, 1930.

9. Dr West/Mrs Gurney 24 December 1841 (recorded in the minutes).

10. Baly, M.E. *Florence Nightingale and the Nursing Legacy*, Croom Helm, London, 1986, Chapter 2.

11. Rathbone, E. *William Rathbone A Memoir*, Macmillan, London, 1904, p. 156.

12. W. Rathbone/A. Clough 6 June 1860 BL, Add.Mss 47595 f.13.

13. F. Nightingale/W. Rathbone 20 June 1860 BL, Add.Mss 47753 f.1–7.

14. Rathbone, W. *A Short History and Description of District Nursing in Liverpool*, Marples, Liverpool, 1898, p. 8.

15. Nightingale, F. *Introduction to the History and Progress of District Nursing*, Macmillan, 1890.

16. Nightingale, F. Introduction to the *Organisation of Nursing in a Large Town* by W. Rathbone, Longman Green, 1865.

17. C. Langton/F.Nightingale 11 January 1869 GLRO HI/ST/NC.69.

18. Annual Report of the Manchester Nurse Training Institution 1867.

19. F. Nightingale/W. Rathbone 22 June 1867, Picton Library E.1310 f.26.

20. W. Rathbone/F. Nightingale 16 June 1874, Picton Library E.1310 f.49.

21. Report of the Sub-Committee for the National Association for Providing Trained Nurses for the Sick Poor, GLRO NC/15/13b, June 1875.

22. Ibid.

23. W. Rathbone/F. Nightingale 17 July 1875, BL, Add.Mss 47754, f.348.

24. *The Times* 14 April 1876, p. 6, col. c.

25. F. Nightingale/H. Bonham Carter 29 January 1875, BL, Add.Mss 47719, f.87.

26. F. Nightingale/W. Rathbone 5 March 1875, BL, Add.Mss 47719, f.42.

2

Founding the Victoria Jubilee Institute

Queens have long been associated with nursing. St Margaret, Queen of Scotland in the eleventh century not only built hospitals but is said to have personally nursed the sick. Her daughter, Maud, wife of Henry I of England carried on the tradition, founding hospitals in London and caring for lepers. In the ensuing reign during the bitter conflict between Stephen and his wife, Matilda, the Queen found time to found religious houses, among which was St Katherine's Hospital by the Tower of London built in 1148 for the repose of the souls of her two children. In 1273 St Katherine's was chartered by Queen Eleanor, widow of Henry II, and again by Queen Philippa, Queen of Edward III when 'the visitation of the sick in the neighbourhood of the hospital' was a duty laid on the corporation, and Philippa decreed that henceforth queens of England should be patrons of St Katherine's Hospital which was handed down with all its estates *reginae Angliae nolio succedentibus.*[1]

The Reformation swept away the masses and the religious foundation but the estates and the patronage remained in the hands of the reigning queen. The nursing of the poor sick in the neighbourhood was forgotten. In 1827, yielding to the pressure of the industrial revolution, the Royal Collegiate Hospital was pulled down to make way for St Katherine's docks, and from the proceeds of this now valuable land a new, neo-Gothic building was erected in Regent's Park and a residence and £1200 was assigned to the master, while six small houses were given to three brothers and three sisters who were in fact recipients of grace and favour for services to the court.

In 1837 the patronage of this institution passed to the young Queen Victoria, who, taking her position seriously, appointed a clerical master. By mid-century, however, reform was in the air and a charity commission was appointed to examine a number of medieval foundations and the purpose to which they were now put. Among them was St Katherine's Hospital. Histories of these foundations were examined, and in a preface to a book on St Katherine's the Duke of Westminster suggested that the now considerable resources of St Katherine's be used for the poor sick in the east part of London for whose inhabitants Queen Philippa had originally intended the services of the hospital.

Once it was known that there were to be new rules for St Katherine's there were a number of applicants in the field. One was the Duke of Westminster himself on behalf of the Metropolitan and National Nursing Association who wanted to extend their work and who claimed that *they* could fulfil the work that Queen Philippa had placed on St Katherine's. The Metropolitan and National needed the money.

There were other claimants, one of which was the East London Nursing Association founded as early as 1868 by the joint efforts of a Mr Robert Wigram and Mrs Stuart Wortley. The East London was an example of amateur control where a 'lady of means' provided lodging and supervised a nurse, acting as her guide and counsellor. In her survey of 1874 Miss Lees condemned the system and the East London,[2] but when the Metropolitan and National Nursing Association was founded the East London Association agreed to amalgamation and Robert Wigram was appointed to the main committee. Contrary to the rules of the Metropolitan and National Association, the East London continued to operate a system of non-resident home nursing and it was soon clear to the watchful Miss Lees that: 'the East London nurses were nothing more than district visitors or mission women, nor was it possible for their District Superintendents to have any control over them'.

A branch Home was eventually established in the Holloway Road, but after the threat of mass resignations by the staff the committee of the Home resigned and Mr Wigram began his campaign against Miss Lees which was to lead to bitterness and recrimination on the main committee.[3] This then was the background to some of Miss Lees' difficulties; it was the clash of two different philosophies. The East London's hat was in the ring to pay off old scores; however, they had one telling shot in their locker: their President was Helena, Princess Christian, a daughter of Queen Victoria, and that, as Miss Nightingale said in another context 'made things awkward'.

While the rival claimants fought for the St Katherine's charity, Queen Victoria, advised by her private secretary, Sir Henry Ponsonby, had other ideas. In 1879 Sir Henry wrote to the Westminster Hospital where the Queen's confidante, Lady Augusta Stanley, had founded a Nurses' Home with the intention of nurses doing 'district visiting', saying that the Queen wished to do certain things to raise the social position of nurses. The Queen proposed that a number of nurses from different institutions should be created 'St Katherine's nurses', and Lady Augusta and the chairman of the Westminster Hospital, Sir Rutherford Alcock, were invited to submit the first three names.[4] Sir Rutherford's early connection with the St Katherine's award and with the Stanleys seems to be the main reason why he was chosen as a trustee of the Queen's Jubilee Institute when it was founded.

The situation at the Westminster Hospital was complicated. In 1873, wanting to reform their nursing services, the governors invited the two Miss Merryweathers to come from Liverpool and supply nurses for the hospital and the district. Mary was the lady superintendent and Elizabeth was the matron. Neither had been trained as nurses although they had visited St Thomas's and Miss Nightingale after a trying day with Mary wrote an exasperated note to Bonham Carter: 'Does she know anything about nursing? She told me nurses fear any stricter discipline than hers . . . her rule at Liverpool has been a failure'.[5] An indication that Miss Nightingale was not in favour of discipline for the sake of discipline. Whatever the cause, the nursing system at Westminster did not work, there were disagreements with the committee and there was no training school until Miss Pyne came from St Thomas's in 1880. Moreover, in order to gain income the home sent out its nurses to private patients as well as to the poor, as had happened in Liverpool and, as Miss Nightingale said in a letter to Mr Rathbone: 'Where private nursing has been combined with district nursing it has ended with district nursing being given up altogether, eg. the Westminster Hospital and its Nurses' Home'.[6]

The new St Katherine's honour to three Westminster nurses did little to forward the cause of district nursing or the sick in their homes in the east end of London. This episode accounts for the misunderstanding about Miss Nightingale's attitude to pensions for nurses.[7] She was in favour of a provident system of pensions for *all* nurses, but she was bitterly opposed to decorations or pensions in lieu of salary as a reward to selected nurses: 'are we not a bit young for the Garter?' she wrote to Henry Bonham Carter.

Although the idea of St Katherine's pensions for a few nurses seems to have fallen through, the possibility of a link between St Katherine's and district nursing continued to be pursued by Sir Henry Ponsonby, and there the matter rested with various claimants — nursing and otherwise — making bids for the St Katherine's charity.

Soon, however, there was a greater prize on the horizon. In 1887 Queen Victoria had been on the throne for 50 years; since Albert's death in 1861 she had retreated into the shadows of widowhood, and now, complaining bitterly of rheumatism, she said she had no wish to face 'an orgy of hustle and bustle', but with the help of the Prince of Wales, face it she did. The women of England were determined to honour the Queen in their own way, committees were set up throughout the kingdom and a head office was opened in Carteret Street, London, with Major Tully as the honorary secretary. The committee was anxious that the offering should be a personal gift to the Queen and, striking an acceptable note, they suggested yet another statue be erected to Prince Albert in Windsor Park. In order to satisfy the donors, a specially designed necklace and earrings were executed by Carringtons of Regent Street, but this still left £70 000 and the Queen had to decide what to do with it. Sir William Jenner, now the Royal physician, suggested a scheme to support emigration, but Sir Henry Ponsonby wanted a committee of advice graced by such women as Florence Nightingale and Mrs Fawcett to 'shield the Queen', and he himself hoped that the money would be used to help nursing. In the end Sir Henry prevailed, 'although not without some screeching between the great Tory and Whig ladies involved'.[8]

The Queen was interested in nursing. She had supported Mrs Fry and had arranged her meeting with the King of Prussia. She had followed Miss Nightingale's career with interest and approval and had invited her to Balmoral where Prince Albert had been impressed by her intelligence. Because of this she had consented to come out of her retirement in 1872 and open the new St Thomas's, and her daughters were all patrons of nursing. On 19 August the Court Circular announced that the Queen had decided to use the surplus money from the Women's Jubilee Offering for the welfare of nursing. Now the claimants for the St Katherine's bounty renewed their efforts and these included the new and controversial British Nurses' Association led by Mrs Bedford Fenwick, with Princess Christian at their head, and who were campaigning for the registration of nurses.

Meanwhile a *Times* leader assumed that the money was to be used: 'to make provision for the nursing of sick women and girls . . . a committee of gentlemen will be requested to advise as to the best mode of giving effect to the design. . . '.[9] Miss Nightingale, on reading her *Times*, wrote to Mr Rathbone in horror: first, that the nursing was to be exclusively for women, and second, that there should be a 'committee of gentlemen to advise', though she said that if he and Henry Bonham Carter were on that committee much of the objection would be obviated. Miss Nightingale was not in the habit of objecting to committees of gentlemen as such, her own Nightingale Council was, and remained, exclusively male, and she never supported the nomination of women in high places. William Rathbone had also seen the announcement in *The Times*, and he sketched out a plan for a district nursing service on a national basis which he sent to Miss Nightingale asking for her opinion and expressing the hope: 'that you will not hesitate to recommend omissions, additions or changes of any kind, I will then, on receipt of your views, and if you think wise, send one copy to the Duke of Westminster'.[10]

Miss Nightingale did send her views, particularly about the training of district nurses and their selection. It is clear that the printed Rathbone plan, which later became the foundation of the Queen Victoria's Jubilee Institute, was the joint effort of himself and Miss Nightingale, though when it comes to the section on the recruitment of nurses: 'There is no doubt that ladies generally make the best district nurses, provided they are sensible and devoted to their work . . . '; they had both been influenced by the strong views of Mrs Craven in insisting on educated gentlewomen — not a view they would have held some 20 years previously.

They saw that district nursing, if it was to raise the standard of hygiene and care in the homes of the poor, required women who were literate and articulate. Whether all Mrs Craven's nurses were ladies is another matter. At one stage during the Holloway fracas Miss Nightingale wrote in exasperation 'they call themselves ladies, give me ward maids!'.[11] But in spite of a few black sheep the idea was put across firmly that the new style of district nurse needed to be better educated and have a longer training than the hospital nurse.

However, Sir Henry Ponsonby was wedded to his scheme for St Katherine's with special decorations and he put up his own plan. He suggested that the St Katherine's Hospital be the headquarters of the new Jubilee Association and that sisters, paid by St Katherine's funds, would work under six unpaid sisters under the patronage of the Queen and the Master. The Chapter would consist of seven ruling sisters, 'two from each kingdom and one from Wales with ruling sisters living in their own departments'. There would also be 30 St Katherine's nurses appointed for 30 years at £30 a year by the Chapter and attached to hospitals, available for duty when ordered by the patron. Nursing associations would join the central association and would probably augment their funds while retaining their own bodies. Sir Henry claimed that what he was aiming at was a sort of 'university of all nursing societies with the Queen at the head granting awards and decorations'.

The scheme, written out in Sir Henry's bold hand, is vague and almost incomprehensible, but it is interesting, as is the scheme submitted by Sir Rutherford Alcock, because both show the wide gap in the thinking of professionals like Miss Nightingale, Mr Rathbone and Mrs Craven, and those around the Court — and indeed elsewhere — who saw reformed nursing, not as a paid profession, but as a pseudo-religious order to be rewarded with decorations and in some cases grace and favour pensions. However, 27 years after the founding of the first Nightingale School the message had still not been put across, namely, that nursing was a secular profession that required a specific training and should be rewarded with an appropriate salary. The Ponsonby plan was seen by Miss Nightingale as anathema. It embodied her *bête noire*, that of making nurses accountable to a chaplain and rewarding them not with pay but with decorations. The revival of medieval customs and institutions may have romantically inspired the nineteenth-century pre-Raphaelites and Tennyson, but they were hardly a foundation for modern scientific nursing.

However, more than the Court were interested in the £70 000. The announcement in *The Times* started a spate of letters; some correspondents disapproved of the scheme claiming that the money was a personal gift to the Queen, but the majority of writers approved and one gives a hint of the social unrest that was being provoked by the economic depression of the time: 'When so much class feeling unfortunately exists, do not alter Her Majesty's intention so happily this Jubilee year spanning the distance between the throne and the cottage . . . '.[12]

A few days later Sir Henry Burdett, the founder of the Hospitals' Association and the owner of the *Nursing Mirror*, weighed in claiming that 'there were 15 000 nurses today of whom a half to two-thirds were certificated'. What was needed, Sir Henry said, was not another nursing organisation, but a Directory of Nurses and a national pension scheme. Sir Henry always exaggerated the number of 'certificated nurses' partly to thwart Mrs Bedford Fenwick and the British Nurses' Association, who were also asking to be considered for money from the Jubilee gift. In fact *The Times* quickly became a vehicle for the various advocates of the different nursing politics of the day. The exhortation to nurses to be 'political' is not new. The nineteenth-century nurses and their patrons pursued their political aims with no holds barred, libel actions not excluded.

The Queen had decreed that the money was going to the nursing of the sick in their own homes and the North London Nursing Association was on safer ground when they wrote giving statistics, and saying that: 'they fulfilled the conditions of the Queen's Bounty except that they were not affiliated, but the Association had worked hard with great success since it was cast adrift seven years ago'.[13] This was a reference to the clash with the iron discipline and standards of Miss Lees in 1880 when the North London had been disaffiliated from the Metropolitan and National Association. Not to be outdone, Mr Wigram wrote on behalf of the East London Nursing Society saying they too 'had been cast off and had resumed work on our old lines . . . our nurses are not the same high class of education but all are hospital trained'.

The letters to *The Times* are interesting because they show that Miss Lees' idea of educated, trained and professionally supervised district nurses was by no means universally acceptable. The supervision of the home nursing of the sick poor, with the exception of the Poor Law, had always been the prerogative of the Church or of the social élite. Change smacked of disturbance in the social fabric, and it says much for William Rathbone that he not only adjusted his own ideas but that he had the skill, the tenacity and the sheer drive to push them through.

In the summer of 1887 William Rathbone's scheme had been printed and sent to the trustees of the fund, who were the Duke of Westminster, Sir Rutherford Alcock and Sir James Paget, who happened to be a friend of Miss Nightingale. The plan was succinct and modelled on his own experience with the Metropolitan and National and his conversion to the idea that the function of almsgiving must be separated from the true task of nursing and health teaching. The paper assumed that the money would not be spent on a building and that the trustees 'should retain, and grant for specific periods, on conditions they should lay down, annual payments to existing institutions'. The point was made, and heavily emphasised, that Queen's nurses should be engaged solely in the services of the poor sick. This was a clause to which Sir Henry Ponsonby objected, and which was to prove a stumbling block to several organisations who supplied nurses for the better-off and who relied on their payments to help with funds for the poor.

The Rathbone/Nightingale scheme was more specific than anything that had been presented before. It laid down a standard of training and selection requirements based on the rules of the Metropolitan and National Nursing Association. It recommended that local Nursing Associations wishing to have trained Queen's nurses should be responsible for their board and lodging expenses and, ultimately, for their salaries. The cost to such an organisation for one nurse was reckoned to be about £80 to £85 a year. Mr Rathbone's paper goes on:

> perhaps the safest course at first would be for the trustees and the committee to take into their confidence the Metropolitan and National Association, giving them a grant for a certain number of years, subject to them giving satisfaction, and employing them to select ladies and train them in London hospitals and in London districts, and to place them out as sanctioned by the executive committee. . . . The trustees might also enquire whether, through other institutions, arrangements could be made for the training for district work nurses of the upper servant class, say in Edinburgh etc.

Mr Rathbone admitted that in hospitals 'training has been given — and as far as I am aware advantageously given — to all classes'. It is significant that Mr Rathbone was now advocating, and apparently with Miss Nightingale's blessing, that in the case of district nurses there should be a special school for officers, something they had set their faces against at St Thomas's ('The lady should be educated with her cook,' said Miss Nightingale). The idea of a school for officers did not last long, but a high proportion of the early Queen's superintendents, to whom the prestige of the Queen's Institute owes so much, were 'Bloomsbury trained'. Miss Nightingale was right when she said 'the Inspectoresses will be all-important'.

During the autumn of 1887 there was much backstairs palace diplomacy and much front stairs to-ing and fro-ing at Miss Nightingale's house in South Street. On 3 November the three trustees met to consider the proposals and to make recommendations. On 5 November Miss Nightingale wrote a long letter to Mr Rathbone saying that she had yesterday received a visit from Sir James Paget who told her that the committee had sent an outline of their scheme to the Queen. The outline consisted of a plan for district nurses to be spread all over the country to affiliate with any existing district nursing associations. The idea of giving salaries only as bare maintenance and making it up with decorations had been totally repudiated. Miss Nightingale went on:

> you see we are not out of the wood, still it is better than I expected, better because Sir Rutherford Alcock's rather wild notions have not come up on the tapis, because the Duke of Westminster seems firm and Sir James seems so eminently sensible, and because the main points on your printed paper, to which of course I did not allude, seem to be adopted.

Miss Nightingale goes on to record her conversation with Sir James about the need for nurses to have pensions based on a provident system, her distrust of certificates, and the great necessity of trained supervisors. Sir James had expressed a hope that the 'thousands of pounds a year of the St Katherine's trust, now spent on non-resident inmates and the six resident ladies who did nothing would be added and utilised by the Jubilee fund'.

On 1 December Sir Rutherford renewed his 'rather wild notion' in which he set forth the urgent need for a district nursing service; but he saw this as being achieved by the revival of the Sisters of St Katherine's with a corps of a 'thousand St Katherine's nurses'. How these were to be selected or trained Sir Rutherford did not say. Miss Nightingale, seeing Sir Rutherford's paper, sent an urgent letter to Mr Rathbone pointing out the dangers of such a scheme.

'How can the East London and Bloomsbury be linked together?' Either one must rise and the other must fall and I am afraid the latter is more likely. If you link together a butterfly and a mole you do not make a bird.[14]

Miss Nightingale apparently did not agree with Voltaire that 'the best is the enemy of the good'. It seems, however, that Sir Rutherford's views did not prevail and that he was subsequently educated to a different view by the Cravens, for on 7 January 1888 the scheme outlined in a letter to *The Times* over his name and the other two trustees was in fact a modification of the Rathbone plan.

We believe that the institution should have its chief centre in London but similar central institutions should be in Edinburgh and Dublin, and that with one, or all of them should be affiliated any institution desiring such affiliation, and satisfactorily fulfilling, in any part of the kingdom, the general purpose of the foundation. We would recommend that the nurses should all be duly approved women of excellent personal character, and of good education, similar to that of well-trained nurses in hospitals, and a special training in district nursing and maternity hospitals, so that they may be fit to attend poor women after childbirth.[15]

In July 1888, the Queen approved the scheme and the trustees transferred the executive part of their duties to a Provisional Committee with the Duke of Westminster as chairman and Mr Rathbone as the honorary secretary. Later Mr Rathbone described this committee as 'the most efficient I have ever known as it seldom met'.[16] Meantime Sir Henry Ponsonby and Sir Rutherford Alcock pursued their enquiries with the Lord Chancellor about the position of St Katherine's Hospital, and the Queen herself was anxious that St Katherine's should be incorporated with the new Jubilee Institute. Once the legal difficulties had been cleared away the master of St Katherine's Community, the Reverend Arthur Lewis Babbington Peile, was made President of the Jubilee Institute, a post which he held for fifteen years and the Queen's Institute started its life in that prestigious neo-Gothic building in Regent's Park. In his history of District Nursing, William Rathbone, ever hopeful, wrote:

> The wasteful system of renewal of leases by fines which formerly existed in the institution has been stopped and it is hoped that when the effect of the system on its income has passed away considerable funds will be available for the Queen's Institute.[17]

Alas, it was not the marriage of true minds; the aims of St Katherine's had little in common with the concept of producing an organisation of professional, well-trained nurses to cover the whole of the United Kingdom, and in the end the Jubilee Institute gained little from its connection with St Katherine's. It is true that it provided accommodation for 'convalescent nurses' after a kitchen had been adapted with pipes from a boiler to fill a tin bath. This was nearly a century after Nelson had had five baths fitted with taps at his house in Merton.

On 20 September 1889, Queen Victoria issued a Royal Charter and the Queen Victoria's Jubilee Institute for Nurses was constituted as a body politic and corporate with a President and Council to take charge of the annual income of the fund and to employ it for the purposes for which Her Majesty intended, namely,

> the training support and maintenance of women to act as nurses for the sick poor and the establishment (if thought proper) of a home or homes for nurses and generally the promotion and provision of improved means of nursing the sick poor.[18]

The following February the Queen appointed a Council consisting of His Grace the Duke of Westminster, Sir James Paget, Sir Rutherford Alcock Trustees; Mrs Theodore Acland, Mrs Dacre Craven, Mrs Henry Grenfell, the Lady O'Hagan, the Hon. Lady Ponsonby, the Countess of Rosebery, Mr Henry Bonham Carter, the Reverend

B. Darley, Sir Dyce Duckworth MD, Oliver Heywood Esq., John Jaffray Esq., the Right Hon. the Earl of Meath, with Mr W. Rathbone as the Vice-President. From this it can be seen that many of the Council were not mere figureheads but had considerable experience with the running of district nursing associations. For the first time in history an eminent Council had a nurse as a member; Mrs Craven no doubt owed her membership to the Queen's extensive corre-spondence with her daughter, Vicky, the Crown Princess of Prussia.

The following month a Scottish Council was appointed with the indefatigable Countess of Rosebery as President, who when she died was replaced by a daughter of the Queen, Her Royal Highness, Princess Louise, the Marchioness of Lorne, thus giving Scotland, a country dear to the Queen, a direct link with royal patronage. In November the Provisional Council made its report to the trustees; in two years much had been accomplished, but as the report pointed out

> Much of this was due to the valuable work of Mr Rathbone, who undertook from the outset the onerous duties of honorary secretary. The efficient manner in which the work devolving on him in that capacity has been carried out for the benefit of the Institute and the promotion of its objects demanded unremitting attention on his part and never failed. Such labours in the initiatory stage have been fully appreciated and cannot be passed over in silence by the Com-mittee, which has so largely profited by his assistance and wide experience in similar work.[19]

There is no doubt but that William Rathbone, in close collabora-tion with Miss Nightingale and Mrs Craven, was the driving force behind the inception of the Queen's Institute and the fact that it finally emerged in a form designed to raise the standard of district nursing, and to meet health needs of a rapidly changing society, was due to his skill, tact and energy.

The fund yielded an annual income of £2049; this would obviously go but a small way towards accomplishing so great a task. Therefore, until such time as the public saw the need for a professional district nursing service and were prepared to pay for it, the Council had to concentrate on producing standards of excellence and pioneering pro-jects that would of themselves educate the public in the need. Several members of the Provisional Council were connected with the Nightingale Fund Council, where the same problem had to be faced, namely, how to make good use of limited resources. The Council eschewed the idea of creating an institution in a new building, but built on, and improved, the existing model, hoping to produce a reformed system of nursing that authorities would soon find it worthwhile to finance for themselves. The Nightingale Fund was merely a grain of mustard seed.[20] The Queen's Institute was to be another mustard seed growth.

In the case of the Jubilee Fund, the Provisional Council built on the Metropolitan and National Nursing Association to which they now gave £450 a year. The Metropolitan and National had been in financial difficulties for some time, and the Queen's bounty saved them and helped them to extend their training with a valuable course of lectures by distinguished professors of medical science, bearing specially on the duties and work of district nurses.

The Provisional Council laid down the Conditions of Affiliation which were:

(1) The standard of training and qualifications of nurses of any association to be affiliated shall be practically the same as that adopted by the Council, in accordance with the Regulations under which Queen's nurses are trained and enrolled.

(2) In order that the same standard of efficiency may be maintained, the Council reserve to themselves the right of requiring reports from the affiliated associations and of periodical inspection of the nurses' work.

(3) The following qualifications shall be considered requisite in order to entitle a nurse to be placed on the roll of Queen's nurses, namely:

    (a) Training at some approved general hospital or infirmary for not less than one year.

    (b) Approved training in district nursing for not less than six months, including the nursing of mothers and their infants after childbirth.

    (c) Nurses in country districts (in accordance with paragraph 8 of these conditions), must have at least three months' approved training in midwifery.

(4) In large towns nurses shall reside in homes, and be under the charge of a trained superintendent approved by the Council.

(5) The nursing of patients shall be conducted under the direction of the medical practitioners.

(6) While not excluding cases of such patients as are able to make some small contribution to the local institution, the services of the nurses are to be strictly confined to the poor.

(7) In towns attendance as a midwife upon women in childbed shall be excluded; but the nursing of mothers and their infants after childbirth may be undertaken when the medical attendant requires the services of a skilled nurse, on condition that proper arrangements can be made for the nurse's other cases.

(8) In country districts the nursing of mothers and their infants may be undertaken whenever required by the circumstances of the patients, but the duties of the midwife, as distinguished from a nurse, are not to be undertaken, except in cases of emergency, or by the express permission of the Local Committee; and with regard to such cases, on condition that proper arrangements and precautions are taken with reference to the nurse's other patients.

(9) The nurses are strictly forbidden to interfere in any way with the religious opinions of the patients or members of their families.

The conditions of affiliation are important, first, because with minor modifications they remained in force for some time and were the backbone of the Institute; second, because failure to comply with some clause or other was the usual reason for disaffiliation in later years. District nursing associations were invited to apply for affiliation and within two years 31 organisations had done so, one of the first being the pioneer association of Liverpool which now had trained nursing superintendents. Some, like the Ranyard Mission, applied in vain, the Queen's Council having decided that their overt religious mission offended against the strict non-sectarian clause in the Charter. Others, though willing, could not afford the cost, and others did not want, or see the need for, Mrs Craven's young ladies of superior education.

In Edinburgh, a Central Institution had been formed and the Scottish Committee took over premises in Charlotte Street as a training home and engaged Miss Peter as their superintendent. Work began in Edinburgh with three nurses where it was required that: 'The Queen Victoria nurses should be highly trained and educated because, although they work under the direction of medical men, these they rarely meet'[21] — a cry latter day Queen's nurses would echo.

The situation in Dublin proved more difficult. A committee was formed with equal numbers of Protestants and Roman Catholics, but it was impossible to carry out a scheme on the same lines as in England and Scotland. The Roman Catholics insisted on separate homes for Catholic and Protestant nurses, and there were other difficulties so that the Provisional Council came to the conclusion that 'the work of nursing the poor in Dublin must be carried out by some of the institutions already in existence in or near the city and the establishment of a new institution was not practical'.

Dublin already had a district nursing association. In 1876, Lady Plunkett, visiting the area around St Patrick's cathedral was shocked at the misery she saw and felt that she should do something to alleviate the distress and she set up St Patrick's Home for District Nurses. In 1881 the Home moved to St Stephen's Green and the nurses were known as 'The Nurses out of the Green'. St Patrick's Home became affiliated to the Queen's Institute, as did St Lawrence's Home which had been established in Parnell Square to cater for the north side of the city. A Council was formed and directed both homes on the principles laid down by the Queen's Institute under the direction of Miss Dunn who had trained at Bloomsbury.[22] However, in spite of these advances the Committee confessed that 'the organisation in Dublin cannot be considered complete'. Dublin was to continue to give Mr Rathbone much anxiety. But considering the sectarian problems, the poverty and the background of the Home Rule Bill, it is a source of wonderment that the scheme, inspired as it was by the British crown, ever came to the remarkable fulfilment that it did. After the First World War when Ireland was torn by strife, the Queen's nurses, north and south, continued sending in their reports to London, visiting, and being visited by, the General Superintendent.

The problem of the Principality of Wales was not religious but linguistic. It was noted that a considerable proportion of the population did not speak English and consequently it was desirable to have a certain number of Welsh-speaking nurses. A public meeting was held in Cardiff and a committee formed to establish a District Nursing Institution which it was hoped would constitute a training centre for Wales.

Mr Rathbone reported:

The Provisional Committee have made a good beginning and laid a firm foundation for future efforts . . . the history of district nursing has reached the commencement of a new chapter in which we believe the consolidation of local efforts into one united royal and national undertaking will mark a new era of its success.[23]

Consolidating local efforts and establishing a national undertaking was a formidable task. That it was eventually achieved was due to the fact that although the aims of the founders were high, the changing social scene, the new awareness of the health needs of the community, together with the greater emancipation and better education of women at the end of the century, brought it within the bounds of possibility. The time was ripe.

NOTES

1. Rathbone, W. *History and Progress of District Nursing*, Macmillan, London, 1890, p. 83.

2. Lees, F. A Report on Hospitals in London 1874/GLRO HI/ST/NC 15, 13a.

3. F. Nightingale/Bonham Carter 22 April 1879, BL Add. Mss 47720, f. 6.

4. Hansell, P. *The Westminster Hospital 1716–1974*, Pitman Medical Press, London, 1974.

5. F. Nightingale/Bonham Carter 25 July 1874, BL Add. Mss 47719, f. 68.

6. F. Nightingale/W. Rathbone 14 August 1887 (copy Queen's Institute).

7. Smith, F.B. *Florence Nightingale: Reputation and Power*, Croom Helm, London, 1982, p. 168.

8. Longford, E. *Victoria RI*, Pan Books, London, 1974, p. 625.

9. *The Times*, 19 August 1887, the leader, p. 7.

10. W. Rathbone/F. Nightingale 23 August 1887, quoted by Zachary Cope, Early History of District Nursing. *Nursing Times* 12 August 1955, p. 886.

11. F. Nightingale/W. Rathbone 11 January 1878, BL Add. Mss 47719, f. 226.

12. *The Times*, 3 September 1887, letter.

13. *The Times*, 21 January 1888, letter from the Treasurer of the North London Nursing Association.

14. F. Nightingale/W. Rathbone 3 December 1888 (copy Queen's Institute).

15. *The Times*, 7 January 1888, letter from the Trustees.

16. Rathbone, E. *A Memoir of William Rathbone*, Macmillan, London, 1905.

17. Rathbone, W. *The History and Progress of District Nursing*, Macmillan, London, 1890, p. 84.

18. The Royal Charter (quoted by Rathbone 1905, pp. 111f.).

19. Westminster, Duke of, Report of the Provisional Committee, 9 November 1889.

20. Baly, M.E. *Florence Nightingale and the Nursing Legacy*, Croom Helm, London, 1986.

21. Report of the Scottish Branch 1890.

22. Crowley, F. *A Century of Service 1880–1980: The Story of the Development of Nursing in Ireland*, 1980, pp. 26–9.

23. Rathbone, W. *The History and Progress of District Nursing*, Macmillan, London, 1890, pp. 88–9.

3

A New Chapter in District Nursing

The first Council of the Queen Victoria's Jubilee Institute for Nurses, appointed by the Queen herself, consisted of 22 members and included Their Royal Highnesses the Princess Christian, the Princess Louise and Princess Beatrice, the three trustees, the Master of St Katherine's as President and William Rathbone as Vice-President. The remaining members were selected from the Provisional Council and were mainly people who had experience in running district nursing associations. In spite of her partiality for Disraeli, Queen Victoria described herself as a 'liberal' and the Council had a distinctly liberal bias. Lady Mary Ponsonby, a friend of the Queen, was well known for her championship of working-class rights and higher education for women, the Countess of Rosebery was the wife of a Liberal peer, Henry Bonham Carter was a Liberal supporter and campaigner for various reform groups, and of course William Rathbone himself was a Liberal MP.

The day-to-day running of the Institute's affairs was conducted from rooms over the Chapter House at St Katherine's in Regent's Park, which were furnished as offices and run by a full-time secretary. In a letter Sir Henry Ponsonby indicated that the Queen had 'approved an early settlement of the position in regard to St Katherine's and that new rules would be referred to the Chancellor'.[1] Sir Henry was hopeful that funds from St Katherine's would augment those of the Jubilee Institute.

THE FIRST INSPECTOR GENERAL: ROSALIND PAGET

The first task of the Executive Committee was to appoint an Inspector General who would be responsible for all nursing matters. This in itself was an innovation. No district nursing association at that time had a nurse to control nurses. After discussion the choice fell on Miss Rosalind Paget, who was a niece of Mr Rathbone and also the niece of the Liberal MP for Bosworth. Partly brought up in the Rathbone household, Rosalind Paget became interested in nursing and social reform. After short spells in Liverpool and Manchester hospitals she spent some time in the Westminster Hospital and then trained at the London Hospital in 1882 under Miss Lückes, a friend of Miss Nightingale, and at that stage Miss Nightingale was looking more favourably on the London Hospital than on St Thomas's.[2] Miss Paget emerged from her training with a glowing report and a reputation for teaching.

From the London Hospital she went to the London Lying-in Hospital and took the certificate of the London Obstetrical Society, which had been established in 1826 and started holding examinations in 1872, and which aspiring midwives were taking, *faute de mieux*, while they pressed for registration.[3] Midwifery was, and remained, Miss Paget's main love and for her contribution to the improvement in the midwifery service she was created a Dame of the British Empire in 1934. In the meantime, at the age of 34 years, in 1890 she accepted an invitation from the Queen's Institute to become the first Inspector General, having first done the district nursing course at Bloomsbury under Miss Mansel. Because of her commitments to her parents, Miss Paget did not use that accommodation provided at St Katherine's but her domestic duties did not deter her from extensive travelling during the two years she held the post. Miss Paget was responsible for all matters relating to the training of nurses, the setting up of schools of district nursing, the granting of certificates and recommendations for enrolment, and the more delicate and difficult task of decisions about affiliation. Under her persuasive and guiding hand, the East London Nursing Association came back into the fold, though with Princess Christian, that active patron of nursing, on both governing bodies it would have been difficult for them to do otherwise. Miss Paget herself took no salary and left in 1891 because of her father's illness, but the Queen appointed her to the Council where she gave valuable advice. Although her professional life was devoted to improving the midwifery services Rosalind Paget never lost her early affection for district nursing and she was a contributor to its journals.

MISS MANSEL AND MISS PETER

Miss Paget was replaced by Miss Mansel from the Metropolitan and National Association, who, like her predecessor, left to marry, yet another Nightingale to 'forsake her work' to be a wife. The third name in the roll of Queen's nurses was that of Miss Pauline Peter, the Superintendent of the Scottish branch, who now transferred to Regent's Park to become the General Superintendent. Miss Peter stayed until 1905 and under her the system of inspection and reporting grew, with regional inspectors sending reports from all over the country, and from those that remain a picture of district nursing at the end of the nineteenth century emerges.[4]

THE UNIFORM AND BADGE COMMITTEE

The main work of the Council devolved on the Executive Committee and through them to subcommittees and one of the most assiduous was the Uniform and Badge Committee. The Queen herself was wedded to the idea of decorations and it was important that the Queen's nurses should look distinctive. After debate it was agreed that the Council would design and recommend a 'Queen's uniform' and then advise the affiliated associations to adopt the design. The committee met in Lady Ponsonby's rooms in St James's Palace almost monthly for 18 months, with Lady Ponsonby as the go-between with the Queen. It was agreed that enrolled Queen's nurses should wear a brassard on the left arm with the Queen's cipher, surmounted by the imperial crown embroidered in gold on a Jubilee ribbon four inches wide. However, this ran into trouble. Converted to the germ theory, the committee said 'what about infection?' Lady Ponsonby agreed to test the proposed brassard in disinfectant, only to find to her horror that the colour turned yellow and the gold black. The brassard was duly modified to dark blue dungaree material. Much thought was given to the badge which was to be worn as a pendant on ribbon round the neck. It was put to the committee that the Queen wished 'to establish some Order in connection with the Institute either by the resuscitation of the Order of St Katherine's or in some other way'.[5] After some diversity of opinion, it was decided that there should be three classes of badge, gold, silver and bronze; the gold and silver badges being suspended on light blue and dark blue ribbon, and the bronze on dark blue cord. With the Queen's approval, the badge itself was designed by Mrs Rathbone and consisted of the Queen's cipher, VRI and the crown, for, having become Empress of India in 1876, Victoria was proud of being Imperial; it kept her up with her nephew William in Prussia whom she disliked. The cipher was inscribed QVI Institute for Nurses 1887. The gold and silver badges were given for distinguished service while the bronze was given to the ordinary Queen's enrolled nurse. All badges declared, or should have declared, that a certain standard of training and efficiency had been obtained. Miss Nightingale maintained that badges, like certificates only proclaimed the standard achieved on the day the nurse was tested; it told the public nothing about the standard or ability of the wearer later. Logic was on Miss Nightingale's side, but she was swimming against the tide. Badges and certificates, more and more elaborate, were to become the vogue in nursing in the early twentieth century.

The Queen herself took an interest in the uniform and Lady Ponsonby went to and fro with patterns; no detail was too small for discussion. In the end dresses of blue and white striped twill with dark blue collars, cuffs and waistbands were approved together with a white or dark blue apron. The cloak was a dark blue material similar to that worn by the Bloomsbury nurses and for the summer there was a waterproof cape which was originally at the instigation of the practical Miss Nightingale. The bonnet was made of black straw, pointed in the front à la Maria Stuart (Mary Queen of Scots) and trimmed with black ribbon, while that cause of so much controversy in the nursing profession, the cap, was to be 'frilled with lace or cambric'. The whole ensemble was undoubtedly very smart, and so it should be for it cost the not inconsiderable sum of £16.4.0, which represented half a year's salary or the whole year's wage of a parlour maid.

However, it was one thing for the Queen to approve, it was another for associations to find the money and even more to persuade nurses to wear the uniform in the approved manner. A not unusual comment in the Inspector's reports in the early years was 'uniform not quite correct' and sometimes there was a more forthright comment such as 'Gampy in appearance'.

TRAINING

The Queen's Council accepted the Metropolitan and National Association as their central training home and subsequent training was modelled on the syllabus there. As the Reverend Dacre Craven said 'the two institutions have become practically amalgamated. Our nurses are spoken of as Queen's nurses and people have become familiar with the application of aid to the Queen's Institute . . . '.[6] There was, however, a new Medical and Sanitary subcommittee, on which sat three eminent doctors and Mrs Craven who analysed the subjects *not* taught to nurses in hospital and which should figure in a district nurse's training. They were sanitary reform, teaching health matters, ventilation, drainage, water supply, diets for the healthy and the sick, the feeding of infants, infectious diseases, monthly nursing of the lying-in woman, the care of newborn infants. The list is interesting because it encapsulates the main causes of mortality in the late nineteenth century when the infant mortality rate was 154 per 1000 live births. The causes of this high death rate and the means of improving it were not taught in general hospitals whose purpose it was to treat, and if possible cure, only the diseases amenable to medicine or surgery at that time. Cures brought donations. In a coda that would be echoed by nurse educators for the next hundred years the committee concluded: 'The chief use of lectures being to enable them [the nurses] to take an intelligent interest in their work and to make them read and think'.[7]

One book the students were requested to read was that excellent manual prepared by Mrs Craven. In the subsequent controversy about nursing education and who should be responsible for it, it is salutary to think that in 1890 a nurse was writing a standard text book for nurses.

Nevertheless, for all their educational aims it appears that theory and practice were often divorced, a complaint that did not cease in 1890. Miss Nightingale wrote that once the nurse was on her district there was little inspection:

> The local committee was not told what the nurse should do, eg to cook and clean on one hand and on the other to give lectures. They don't even know their own work . . . the nurses write to their inspectors to remonstrate and are told there can be no interference with the local committee. There is no other reason for putting a nurse who has just finished her training somewhere other than that so and so wants a nurse, to have *their* [the nurses] wishes attended to seems unthought of . . . [8].

It is not clear from whom Miss Nightingale got her information, but she was corresponding closely with Miss Amy Hughes, a Nightingale nurse at that time in charge of the Metropolitan and National Association who probably felt that her teaching was not being put into practice. Not for the last time in history was there a rift between the educational needs of the nurse and the practical demands of the service.

AFFILIATION

Perhaps the most hard-pressed of committees was the Affiliation Committee whose records are a long saga of applications for affiliation, some of which are turned down because they do not meet the requirements of the Institute, some turn themselves down because they cannot find the money but want a grant that the Institute cannot afford. Others, having been affiliated become disaffiliated because the Queen's nurse has left and has been replaced by a non-Queen's nurse, or for some reason have 'returned to their old ways'. Not everyone was impressed by the Queen's cipher and some resented interference. It is clear from the minutes that at times the problem lay with the local doctors, who by no means all welcomed the new style of nurse. One local committee to take exception wrote in threatening terms: '. . . a very strong feeling against the Queen's Institute [exists] so much that it objected to a Superintendent sending it a Queen's nurse . . . . If the Queen's inspector visited I am afraid she would not be well received . . . '[9]. However, thanks to a diligent Council who always, it seems, had friends and relations among the squirearchy and the nobility who ran the local associations and the tact of the inspectors, progress was made and the number of affiliations grew.

Scotland

In Scotland the branch under its own Council made an energetic start with a training school in Edinburgh. Miss Guthrie Wright, an original member of the council, was the first secretary and during the first year the Edinburgh Queen's nurses paid 7517 visits to 321 cases and a nursing association was set up in Dundee. In Glasgow there was already a Sick Poor and Private Nursing Association which had been founded by Mrs Mary Higginbotham in 1875 and was the pioneer of district nursing in Scotland. In 1889 Glasgow amended its rules and became affiliated to the Queen's Institute; soon it had a Nurses' Home and fourteen nurses in training. By 1891 there were twelve local associations affiliated to the Queen's Institute and the demand for nurses outstripped the supply. The same year the Scottish Council struck an independent note and passed a resolution that they should have the power 'to affiliate such branches from their commencement in a higher standard of local arrangement, this being subject to inspection'.[10] That the Scottish Council had its way was no doubt due to the active interest taken in district nursing by its President, Princess Louise. By the time of the Diamond Jubilee there were 187 Queen's nurses, 69 of whom were able to go to the reception at Windsor.

Ireland

In Ireland there had been long and intense negotiations between the Archbishop of Dublin and Mr and Mrs Rathbone and it was admitted that the Protestant St Patrick's Home, now run by Miss Hunt from Bloomsbury, was the only organisation that gave a training to district nurses. The Archbishop, having had his fears allayed as to the proselytising intentions of the Queen's nurses, agreed to a Joint Committee for District Nursing in Dublin, provided that the domestic life of the Protestant and Catholic nurses was kept distinct, and he had no objection to Catholic nurses working under a Protestant superintendent. Miss Dunn from England with supreme tact trod through this sectarian minefield with such success that when Miss Paget visited Dublin in 1891 her report was full of praise for the quality of training in the Irish Branch and in the following year St Lawrence's Catholic Home was affiliated to the Institute.

But Dublin was not Ireland. Ireland was desperately poor. It had not recovered from the great famine of the 1840s when the population fell from eight million to six million, when half a million died of outright starvation or of disease on ships to inhospitable ports abroad.[11] Unrest, eviction and agrarian outrage produced the Fenians and the bitter struggles of the land league, and at the time of the founding of the Irish Branch the British government and an indignant Queen were reeling from the Phoenix Park murders and there was bitter controversy over the Home Rule for Ireland Bill.

In 1903 Lady Dudley, the wife of the Lord Lieutenant, started a scheme for the establishment of district nurses in the poorest parts of Ireland in the extreme west known as the 'congested areas' where it was difficult to form local committees. In two years enough money was collected to provide nine nurses and the fate of the nurse on Achill island, her cottage and its repairs gave rise to a number of urgent Council minutes. The first *Queen's Nurses' Magazine* in 1904 contains colourful articles of what pioneering district nursing was like in the west of Ireland at the turn of the century. The nurse in Connemara had to walk two miles off the road through bogs to get to patients' cabins where she coped with maternity cases with the cow in the same room or where the tide came through the house; often there was no bed for the patient, no fire because the peat was too wet and the only food potatoes three times a day. Her colleague writes of difficulties due to superstition where it was thought 'if a sick person was washed and his bed made he will do no good', because when washed the patient looked as if he were laid out. Illness was due to the faeries' revenge and a sign that they were stealing the patient away. After dealing with the patient, and presumably the faeries, the nurse mounted her bicycle and started her lonely ride of perhaps eight or nine miles through bog and mountains.[12]

Nevertheless, in spite of the difficulties and the appalling poverty both nurses were impressed with the quiet courtesy and warm welcome of the Irish people and both reported on the support given by the priests. The parish priest at Glengarriff was in accord with Mr Rathbone when he said of the district nurse 'her influence for good is not only confined to the homes of the sick, her example is educating and refining the whole district'.[13] The poor saw the nurse as one who brought comfort, the better off saw her as a moral agent.

By 1904 the Irish Branch had two training schools in Dublin and a third in Londonderry and was training both Protestant and Catholic nurses in harmony; a reminder, if one were needed, that when it comes to sectarian strife, history is not a straightforward progression to the light. From the priests in west Ireland to the parishes of London, people in general, though not always the doctors, welcomed the new style of district nurse. She came at the time of the validation of the germ theory and new ideas on the prevention of ill health, she brought succour to the poor, and, it was argued, saved the poor-rate by returning the sick poor to work.

RAISING MONEY

But it all cost money, and the income from the Jubilee fund was only £2120. By 1893 the expenditure on office administration, salaries and training was £4970 and a subcommittee consisting of Henry Bonham Carter and William Rathbone was set up to make recommendations. The immediate situation had been saved by a gift of £1000 from Mr Rathbone and £5000 from Sir Henry Tate, but this was capital and already £2000 had been spent. A further benefaction from the Berridge Trust was earmarked for teaching and training but this fell short of what was needed, although the committee noted hopefully 'that expenditure on training would decrease as affiliated associations are able to train themselves'. But even with that pious hope the Council needed at least another £2500 a year as permanent income if they were to meet the current commitment.

One way of raising money would have been to extend the appeal. The subject was broached but the Queen, through Sir Henry Ponsonby, decreed that she would 'object to an appeal in her name, or in that of her Council'. The next hope was money from St Katherine's, but although there is correspondence from the Lord Chancellor no money was forthcoming. The committee set in train a number of individual appeals to the public, but the response was poor. During the great depression of 1873–96, with unemployment at times reaching 10 per cent, there were other calls on the public purse and, more important, less profit was being made from which big donations might come.

Fortunately the immediate situation was saved by the Queen's Diamond Jubilee. In 1897 the Queen would have ruled for 60 years — longer than any monarch in Europe — and had emerged from her seclusion to become a popular figurehead. She was the head of a great Empire, threats of abdication had passed, and after the retirement of Gladstone comparative peace reigned between the Queen and her ministers; it was a period of jingoism, the country was at peace before the Boer War and it celebrated accordingly. A Queen's Commemorative Fund Committee was set up under the Duke of Westminster, and what better cause for the money than the Queen's nurses, who, thanks to the public relations efforts of the Council were becoming well known? As in 1887, committees were set up throughout the kingdom and between them they raised £68 000; £48 000 for the extension of the work in England, £19 000 collected in Ireland was invested for work in that country, and £11 000 collected in Scotland was returned to the Scottish Council. A widespread appeal for annual subscriptions followed, resulting in an increase of about £2000 a year to the annual income of the Institute.

The year before the Diamond Jubilee the Queen received nearly 400 of the 529 nurses on the Queen's Roll at Windsor Castle which was duly reported in *The Times* but was more fully and colourfully described by Mr Rathbone in a letter:

the nurses were marshalled four abreast and marched up to the Castle to the private terrace and round the semi-circular garden to the marquee where they had a good substantial lunch. At 5 o'clock they were assembled for inspection by the Queen who was flanked by the Council and many notables of Society. The Queen in an aside said 'they are a very nice looking set' and then made her speech 'I am very pleased to see my nurses here today, to hear of the good work they are doing and I am sure will continue to do'.[14]

Queen Victoria did not make long speeches. It was from all accounts, a great day, not only for the nurses but for the elite of society, and that was good publicity.

In 1901 Queen Victoria died and the Women's Memorial to the Queen was inaugurated to supplement the endowment to the Queen's Institute. By now the Duke of Westminster had died and the committee headed by the Duke of Portland worked unceasingly through the difficulties of the Boer War and in the end £84 000 was added to the endowment. This was helpful but it was still not enough to finance the rapidly expanding work and the Council's aim to promote a universal service of 'thoroughly trained district nurses to cover the whole kingdom'. If they were to attract the right calibre nurses, they had to pay them at least as well as ward sisters in a good hospital and to see that they were housed and cared for properly. Local associations did not always see this need.

Of the money raised in 1897 £5000 was put aside to create a fund for the personal benefit of Queen's nurses and to augment the salaries of the nurses with the longest service; later the fund was added to by Amy, Lady Tate, in memory of Sir Henry who had been a benefactor of the Institute. However, splendid though these efforts were, they did not get to the heart of the matter. Was this to be a service exclusively for the poor sick to be paid for by charitable donations from the better off? Or should it be a service for everyone who could not afford a private nurse but who could, and maybe would, pay towards the cost?

Not everyone approved of a charitable service to the sick poor. The great Victorian virtue was thrift and saving for a rainy day; charity encouraged recklessness. In 1898 Dr Hurry published his book *District Nursing on a Provident Basis*, dedicated to that arch-protagonist of self-help, Octavia Hill. Breathing the spirit of Samual Smiles, Dr Hurry traces the history of district nursing and particularly that of the Queen's Institute and quotes Burdett's *Hospitals and Charities* to show that the Queen's Institute now had 299 affiliated centres with an increasing number of visits being paid to the poor: 'the need is an immense one and no merely charitable movement can supply it'. Referring to the survey by Charles Booth,[15] he points out that 82 per cent of the population were working class and when ill they could not afford a nurse. Hospital accommodation was limited and in any case: 'many illnesses are inadmissible . . . chronic phthises, paralysis, advanced cases of cancer, incurable ulcers, long standing rheumatism . . . '. For the really destitute, Dr Hurry argued, there was the Poor Law, but this invoked the evils of pauperism whereas the district nurse, if well trained, not only saved the poor-rate, but also the hard-pressed hospital and returned the breadwinner to the economy. The district nurse therefore had an economic value.

> Unhappily Institutes of District Nursing, with a few exceptions have been established on a charitable basis and depend almost exclusively on the donations and subscriptions of the upper and middle classes. Hence instead of increasing the independence and self reliance of those to whom the nurse is sent, they exert the opposite effect and encourage them to depend on the gratuitous help of the benevolent . . . There is no more reason why skilled service should be given in the form of free nursing than in the form of free medical attendance.

Strong words, but Dr Hurry was not alone in his contention, though one suspects that some of his fear was not because the Queen's nurses were demoralising the poor but because they were giving advice and treatment free for which, in Dr Hurry's eyes, the patient should have paid a doctor.

The rest of the book is devoted to schemes for organising district nursing on a Provident basis whereby 'a small payment is made in advance, monthly or weekly, to be fixed at a rate so low as to be in the means of all who are not entirely indigent. It is a matter of experience that one nurse is ample for 4,000 persons.' Whose experience Dr Hurry does not say. On that reasoning a scheme of a shilling a year would pay for a district nurse. The book quotes people in favour of a Provident scheme and these include Mr Rathbone himself, Miss Twining and Miss Amy Hughes. It is true they did, but they faced the dilemma that was to beset the Institute for years. Firstly, it was founded as a service to the poor sick and Queen Victoria herself was very conscious of the needs of her poorest subjects. However more important was the fact that Dr Hurry had failed to study the Booth's Survey from which he so tendentiously quoted. Booth had shown that one-third of the population were living below the 'poverty line', and he highlighted the fact that the problems of casual labour, unemployment and old age were beyond private charity or Samuel Smiles self-help, but required state intervention. But state intervention is something of which Dr Hurry would not have approved — nor, indeed, would Queen Victoria.

The problem for the Institute was that probably one-third of the population could not pay a regular subscription. For them there was no old age pension and no dole and that third was in the greatest need of health care, and still are.[16] Moreover, if failure to pay was because the father was feckless, were the family to be denied nursing care? Above all, how was the subscription to be collected? In prosperous industrial areas where an employer was willing to collect from the work force, this was possible. Dr Hurry shows how 9000 workmen in Stockton-on-Tees had subscribed £440 to the Nursing Association, but by no means all workers were so well organised, and what about rural areas? The Institute was firm, and rightly so, that the nurse should not be responsible for collecting money for that would have created an undesirable cash nexus between the patient and the nurse. Eventually, as the service spread, the Institute came round more and more to the idea of collecting subscriptions, but thanks to Victorian poverty and inter-war unemployment voluntary subscriptions were only a partial answer to the financial problems.

Dr Hurry and those who felt like him asked the wrong question, which should have been: why was it in a growing affluent society that perhaps one-third of the population could not afford to make some provision for sickness and old age? The dilemma could not be solved by charity or self-help, but by a state insurance system that would entitle all citizens to at least basic health care. But if the state decided that all classes had a right to some care, then sooner or later the state must pay for the provision of that care. Until that day dawned the Queen's nurses provided a nursing service financed as best it could from donations from the better off, subscriptions from patients willing to pay and soon payments from the state whenever they could get them.

BEGINNINGS OF SCHOOL NURSING

By the end of the century there were 900 Queen's nurses on the Roll and they were expanding their work. In 1891 Amy Hughes at Bloomsbury started a system of school nursing at the Vere Street Board School Board: 'A nurse visited the school every morning and spent between one and two hours seeing 20–40 children and dealing with burns, cuts, abscesses, ophthalmia etc. as well as examining them for dirt and vermin.' Mrs Leon, a school manager, maintained that the nurse improved the attendance because the children had their sores attended to there instead of staying away; she also prevented much pain and discomfort and the spread of infectious diseases.[17] Liverpool, under the enthusiastic guidance of Mrs Rathbone, was quick to follow up the idea and a scheme was started in March 1895, and by the end of the year over 1000 children had been seen.

The Queen's nurses, by a remarkable piece of initiative, had highlighted a crying social need that was soon to be made all too manifest. The Education Act of 1870 had made provision for 'Board Schools' in areas where there were no voluntary schools, but 30 years later it was clear that pupils were not profiting from education because of ill health. The disclosures of the army recruiting office at the time of the Boer War showed that 40–60 per cent of the recruits were rejected on physical defects. The report of the committee set up to enquire into this scandalous state was, amongst other things, to recommend a school health service. However, by the time legislation was enacted the Queen's Institute had already shown the way.[18]

BEGINNINGS OF HEALTH VISITING

Another development at the end of the nineteenth century was the idea that there should be a separate corps of workers trained as 'health visitors'. Since the introduction of Medical Officers of Health a number of cities had employed women as 'health missioners' but none had been trained. In 1891, Miss Nightingale saw the opportunity for training under the new Local Government Act with its provision of technical colleges. She accordingly wrote to her nephew, Frederick Verney, who was conveniently on the council of North Bucks.

I have been making assiduous enquiries for educated women trained in such a way that they could personally bring their knowledge home to cottagers' wives on a mission of health in rural districts. For this they must be *in touch and in love*, so to speak with the rural poor mothers and girls and know how to show them better things without giving offence.

We have, tho' they be but a sprinkling, in one or two great towns and in London excellent Town District Nurses but for obvious reasons they would not be suitable for your proposed work. . . . It hardly seems necessary to contrast sick nursing with this. The needs are quite different; Home Health bringing requires different, but not lower, tho' apparently humbler qualifications and more varied. They require tact and judgement unlimited to prevent the work being regarded as interference and becoming unpopular. They require initiative and real belief in sanitation and that Life or Death may lie in a grain of dust or drop of water or other such minutiae which are not minutiae but Goliaths and the Health Missioner must be David and slay them. She must make her work acceptable to the labouring class.[19]

These words have not lost their force 90 years later though death may lie in different minutiae.

Frederick Verney used his influence and a course for health visitors was planned: 'the health visitor has not the training of the nurse and does not pretend to be one', he wrote.[20] But the idea soon attracted nurses who were realising that much of their work was concerned with dealing with preventable illness. As time went by nurses, women doctors and university graduates saw health visiting as a worthwhile career. The concept of a special training in preventive medicine was soon fostered by the new legislation of the twentieth century, and in 1907 Bedford College and then Battersea College were offering courses for health visitors.

But the district nurse was taught to see herself as a sanitary missionary; improving the health of the family and the environment of the home was Florence Lees' most cherished ideal and to some extent the work overlapped. However, as demands for actual home nursing increased, and the case studies of the early district nurses show this to be so, and new legislation placed more duties on both health visitors and nurses some division of duties seemed inevitable. As Miss Lückes said in another context 'it is a waste to train all for everything'. Whether a nursing qualification based on an acute general hospital should have become the basis for health visiting is debatable. Had the health visitor developed as Miss Nightingale intended, she might all the sooner have been prepared as the general purpose family visitor so needed in the second half of the twentieth century; as it was, both services developed to meet the needs of the early part of the century.

For the district nurse it was the poor sick, often living in slums and below the poverty line; for the health visitor it was soon to be a concentration on the needs of mothers and babies and a campaign to reduce the infant mortality rate, a concentration that led to the idea that nursing and midwifery qualifications were the best basis for the new career of health visiting. In the short term this was successful, but it was at the expense of the original function of the health visitor.[21]

Thus, within a few years district nurses and health visitors were likely to come from the same background of nurse training, one concentrating on home nursing and one on health teaching and this sometimes led to rivalry and misunderstanding which was exacerbated once health visitors were employed and paid by local authorities and the communication gap grew wider.

However, this was in the future. At the beginning of the twentieth century the district nurse had developed as the home nurse, the school nurse and the sanitary missionary, but she was struggling against unequal odds. The needs were overwhelming and the workers were few.

NOTES

1. H. Ponsonby/A.L.B. Peile 3 March 1890, QNI.
2. Baly, M.E. *Florence Nightingale and the Nursing Legacy*, Croom Helm, London, 1986, Chapter 11.
3. Donnison, J. *Midwives and Medical Men*, Heinemann, London, 1977, p. 81.
4. Selected reports from 1897 Public Record Office, PRO 30.
5. Uniform and Badge Committee Minutes 8 July 1890, QNI.
6. Dacre Craven/Duke of Westminster 6 May 1898, QNI.
7. Medical and Nursing Subcommittee Minutes July 1890.
8. F. Nightingale/H. Bonham Carter, undated April 1895, BL Add.Mss 47726, f. 158.
9. S. Martin/Mrs Byron 13 July 1901, QNI.
10. Statements with regard to the position of the Scottish Council, 1891 Report.
11. Webb, R.K. *Modern England*, Allen and Unwin, London, 1969, p. 274.
12. *Queen's Nurses' Magazine*, 31 December 1904, p. 65.
13. *Queen's Nurses' Magazine*, 1 May 1904, p. 17.
14. Rathbone, W. A memorandum quoting Hardy, G. *William Rathbone and Early District Nursing*, G.W. and A. Hesketh, Ormskirk, 1890 p. 24.
15. Booth, C. *Life and Labour of the People of London*, Macmillan, London, 1901.
16. Black, D., Morris, J.N., Smith, C., Townsend, P. *Inequalities in Health: Report of a Research Working Group*, HMSO, London, 1980.
17. Mrs Leon/Mrs Rathbone January 1894, *A Report on Vere St Board School Nursing.*
18. *The Report of the Interdepartmental Committee on Physical Deterioration*, HMSO, 1904.
19. F. Nightingale/F. Verney 17 October 1891, BL Add.Mss 59786, f. 93.
20. Verney, F. Report to the North Bucks County Council, 1892.
21. Clark, J. *A Family Visitor*, RCN publication, 1973, pp. 12f.

4

Rural District Nursing

When the great controversy about the need to reform the old Poor Law was at its height at the beginning of the nineteenth century, eminent clergymen wrote tracts advising a return to the Elizabethan concept of separating the impotent poor from the idle sturdy. The latter, it was argued, should be put to work and not given support from the rates. Government or parish interference was an anathema, not only because it destroyed the incentive to self-help, but because it removed the responsibility from the rich to help the poor.[1] Bearing in mind the teaching about the rich man's difficulty in entering the kingdom of heaven, they pointed out that one passage through the eye of the needle was by charity. If the incentive to charity was removed, the better off would lose their sense of responsibility. The dutiful children sang:[2]

> The rich man in his castle
> The poor man at his gate
> God made them high and lowly
> And ordered their estate.

With the growth of evangelism and bourgeois morality, the Victorian social philosophy crystallised into four great tenets: work, thrift, respectability and self-help. Work was the most useful thing and it had to be practised no matter what your talents or station in life. But running alongside this emphasis on self-help, and in some ways contradictory to it, was the growing awareness of poverty that no amount of thrift or an increase in philanthropy would avert. There was an impressive growth in the number of charities, and in 1861 when the Charity Organisation Society was set up it was estimated that there were no fewer than 640 charitable institutions, many of them concerned with trying to bridge the gap between the 'two nations' by personal contact and by visiting the poor and needy in their own homes.[3]

The other impetus to charitable work was the urge to evangelism in all denominations, but especially by the non-conformists. As Major Barbara said, 'I can't talk religion to a man with bodily hunger in his eyes'.[4] However, some radical reformers like John Stuart Mill, and indeed his disciple Miss Nightingale, realised that in the new industrial towns unemployment and poverty were such that they could not be dealt with effectively by the haphazard agency of charity or the new Poor Law, and they argued in favour of some kind of state intervention. Such arguments were looked at askance by the orthodox utilitarians, who believed in the economic policy of *laissez-faire*, and also by the charity organisations who believed in the personal nexus between the giver and the receiver which was held to be an advantage to both.

The country districts, however, were different. In the latter part of the nineteenth century over 50 per cent of employed females were in domestic service,[5] and there was a close link between the Big House and the cottages at the gate. Many ladies of the manor, or indeed lesser establishments, visited the sick and needy, either from a sense of Christian duty or because the *mores* of society dictated it. As medicine became more respectable, and as the value of nursing became more apparent, particularly after the Nightingale reforms, so ladies began to employ nurses for their poor sick and then to band together and form 'associations'. This ethos of Victorian charitable visiting with its sturdy neighbourhood idiosyncrasies and independence is the heritage of rural district nursing. It is important to remember that with the advent of the Queen's training no new empire was carved out, merely that the new style district nurse was grafted on to the old with all the problems that fusion was to entail.

EARLY RURAL NURSING

In a delightful diary kept by Lady Georgina Vernon of Hanbury between 1869 and 1875, we get a picture of what rural nursing was like before Miss Lees' 'thoroughly trained ladies' started to take over.[6] Lady Georgina visited the patients on her estate with her nurse, who was presumably the village nurse-midwife, because it is recorded that she attended eleven confinements in five months, and would have been the type of midwife for whom the Nightingale training for midwives at King's College Hospital was aimed at that time.[7] Alas, there is no evidence that Lady Georgina availed herself of this opportunity for her nurse-midwife. Apart from midwifery, the diary is a long saga of taking rabbit or cod liver oil to patients: 'took wine for Mrs Wardle's child suffering from abscesses.' Here one is not sure whether the wine is to be used as a dressing or the child was given wine to ease the pain. There seems to be little or no coopera- tion with a doctor, probably the patients were too poor to afford one. A sad entry is 'visited Mrs Bradley's baby and found it dead of inflam- mation of the lungs'. Presumably no doctor was called, and like all too many babies it died from pneumonia, probably induced by poor hygiene and the mother's malnutrition. No amount of wine or rabbit would avail. A tantalising entry reads 'an accident to a cottage from a train'. Lady Georgina does not expound how the accident happened: did it run off the rails? But it is a reminder that the new railway age brought its casualties as well as its benefits.

Elizabeth Malleson

Because of its connection with the Court, it is customary to think of the Queen's Institute as being associated with traditional establish- ment figures, but in fact many who supported the idea of a gratuitous district nursing force were strong-minded women with decidedly radical views. One such figure is Elizabeth Malleson, the original founder of the Rural District Nursing Association, who is noteworthy, not only because of her interest in district nursing, but as an example of how interconnected were the reforming, liberal women of the mid- nineteenth century. They had the leisure, they had the will, they wrote copiously and they knew one another. Born in 1828 into a family steeped in radical politics, Elizabeth Whitehead became a friend of Octavia Hill, the housing reformer, Barbara Leigh-Smith, a women's rights campaigner and Miss Nightingale's cousin, and George Eliot, and she knew and corresponded with Harriet Martineau, whose formidable journalism was the scourge of the reactionaries and male chauvinism. Thus influenced, she decided to help run a school in Lisson Grove for 'children of all classes'. In 1856 Elizabeth married Frank Malleson who shared her interests and together they became associated with Fredrick Denison Maurice, the Professor of Moral Philosophy at Queen's College, London, the leader of the Christian Socialists and the prototype of Shaw's Reverend Morell in *Candida*. In fact Mrs Malleson herself is very much a Shavian woman.

Imbued with neo-socialist ideas, the Mallesons ran a college for working women, where the teachers included Dr Elizabeth Garrett Anderson, William Morris and Octavia Hill, and where they knew all the figures associated with the women's emancipation movement. However, Elizabeth Malleson was a Victorian, and perhaps the victim of Victorian medicine, for after the birth of her fourth child like her friends Harriet Martineau and Miss Nightingale, she took to her bed or her couch. For the sake of her health, the family moved to Dixton Manor in Gloucestershire, where Frank managed the farm and became a member of the County Council and interested himself in the education of the villagers by starting a library and opening the Gotherington Village Hall run on democratic lines.

Mrs Malleson, apparently cured of her invalidism, took an interest in the village, where she was appalled by the high infant mortality rate and where maternal deaths occurred because a doctor was not called. She herself acquired what knowledge she could, and in 1884 started a scheme to raise funds to establish a trained nurse and midwife in the village with the local doctor acting as treasurer. It is a testimony to the strong personalities of the Mallesons that they were accepted as leaders in this conservative community since their politics were socialist, they never went to church and actually played tennis on Sundays. However, the scheme for a trained district nurse ran into trouble. Some saw the scheme as dangerous socialism; the poor, it was argued, would be sapped of vitality if responsibility for their own welfare was taken from them. Mrs Malleson was determined and enlisted the help of her neighbour, Lady Hicks-Beach at Winchcombe, and together they drew up a prospectus for a scheme which was headed by Florence Nightingale and Mrs Dacre Craven and thus was born the Rural District Nursing Association.

THE RURAL DISTRICT NURSING ASSOCIATION

By 1885 the scheme had spread beyond Gloucestershire to other counties, and a central committee was formed which met in no. 11 Downing Street, with Princess May of Teck present. Presumably this was by permission of Sir Michael Hicks-Beach, who was Chancellor of the Exchequer, and who, himself, happened to be a friend of Miss Nightingale and interested in nursing. The aims of the Association were to collect money, to train nurses for district work and to put out publicity material. Each county was encouraged to form a committee, under which were to be grouped district nursing associations with their own management committees. The central committee issued leaflets with advice about pay and conditions for nurses and encouraged affiliation to the Rural District Nursing Association provided that certain conditions were met. These were that only trained nurses and midwives should be recognised as district nurses — a clause that was to prove a stumbling block to some associations, the nurse was to have her own cottage or lodgings and was to be a 'visiting nurse', *living in was to be discouraged*, and except for midwifery cases the services of the district nurse were to be gratuitous, the money being found from donations and offerings from patients.[8]

The principles of the Rural District Nursing Association are important because they run parallel to those laid down by Mrs Dacre Craven for London, and they remained the basic foundation of rural district nursing for many years to come. The Rural District Nursing Association was a flourishing organisation by the time the Queen Victoria's Jubilee Institute was established; within seven years it had eleven county associations with 34 nurses employed who were subject to inspection. With the establishment of the Queen's Institute, it was inevitable that some of the people associated with it and its council members would be those already concerned with the Rural District Nursing Association, and the same names tend to recur, like the Countess of Selborne, the honorary secretary of the Hampshire Association, Lady Victoria Lambton and Lady Susan Gilmour. In 1890 the Rural Association applied for, and was granted, affiliation to the Queen's Institute as the Queen Victoria's Jubilee Institute for Nurses Rural District Branch, and by 1897 there was complete amalgamation and the Rural District Branch ceased to exist as a separate body.

The joining together of two organisations having different origins and very powerful management committees but similar principles helps to explain the complicated structure of the Queen's Institute in the early days; there were many vested interests to be placated and the Queen's Institute Council had to tread a minefield of local pride and prejudice.

The arrangements in Gotherington, Mrs Malleson's own district, give some idea of how the fusion was effected. In 1885 a nurse-midwife was employed with a salary of £1 a week; but the nurse had to wear down the suspicion of the local inhabitants and the doctors before she was accepted. The next nurse was sent to the Radcliffe Hospital for training and when she returned she was supplied with a uniform costing £1.11.6 and, interestingly enough, instruments and dressings costing 15 shillings, which seems to indicate that in spite of medical hostility Mrs Catterell was able to attend some surgical cases. Her method of transport to the distant parts of her district was by donkey and cart, which was apparently cheap and efficient. In 1892, after the amalgamation, a Nurse Garrett succeeded Mrs Catterell, and after being visited by the Queen's Inspector was placed on the Roll of Queen's Nurses and wore the badge and brassard. She was, of course, employed by the Gotherington District Nursing Association. The work grew, the idea of a trained nurse visiting homes was accepted, and two donkeys had to be employed; then sadly, 'the nurse was stricken with illness in the midst of her work' and died, reminding us that infection was a constant occupational hazard of the early district nurses. By 1906 the method of transport had become a bicycle and the Queen's Inspector decided that the district needed two nurses. By now Gotherington was affiliated to the Gloucestershire County Nursing Association and the nurses were under the surveillance of the County Superintendent. Gotherington encapsulates the story of from handywoman-midwife to Queen's trained nurse in a span of 20 years, which must have been typical of many rural areas.

RURAL MIDWIFERY

But the transition was not always smooth. In 1902 the Midwives Act required a certificated midwife to attend every case. After a bitter struggle with the medical profession and a series of abortive parliamentary bills between 1890 and 1900, the Central Midwives Board had been set up which ensured a minimum of three months' training, soon becoming longer, and the conferment of a certificate by examination.[9] This meant that County Nursing Associations had to undertake to supply an increased number of midwives. But midwifery is always an uncertain business. A midwife with rural duties could only cover a limited area because of distance. Donkeys or even bicycles could only go so fast, and only part of her time could be used for midwifery. In practice, the midwife was called on by the whole population for advice about families and for assistance in the case of sickness. But the midwife was not trained as a nurse, and at that time it was impossible to obtain sufficient numbers who were trained. Professor Abel-Smith has calculated that by 1901 there were only 10 000 trained to a standard that would have satisfied either Florence Nightingale or Mrs Bedford Fenwick,[10] and these were needed in hospitals and the growing, and more attractive, demands for private nursing. It was the heyday of the Private Nursing Association and comparatively few trained nurses were available for district nursing. In the circumstances the Institute had to come to terms with a compromise between what was possible and what was desirable — a conflict that was to face the nursing profession for many years to come.

To meet the need of the village nurse-midwife who was not a trained nurse, a special training was organised at the Plaistow Maternity Charity and District Nurses' Home in the east of London and which had been set up for rescue work. The Council of the Queen's Institute spent much time discussing this scheme, for the Home was imbued with the philosophy of the Charity Organisation Society, and it was feared that the training would concentrate too much on welfare and not enough on nursing. In 1896 an experiment was started in Lincolnshire by Lady Warwick whereby the District Nursing Association employed village nurse-midwives under the aegis of the Queen's nurses. Mr Rathbone, writing to Miss Peter, says he had discussed this scheme with Henry Bonham Carter and they were agreed that the matter must be brought to a head and, while looking to the day 'when all areas will be served by thoroughly trained Queen's nurses', they enunciated two principles that must be observed:

> that only nurses with a thorough hospital and district training can be Queen's nurses in accordance with the rules. Any district affiliated and inspected where Plaistow nurse-midwives are employed, other than duly accepted Queen's nurses [the nurses] shall be described by a name that distinctly marks the difference between them.[11]

Here the Council hit upon two difficulties: what was a 'thorough training', and was it measured in length? The Nightingale training was still officially one year, though by now most probationers were working their three-year contract with the Nightingale Fund at St Thomas's Hospital.[12] The other difficulty was over the title 'nurse' which was to beset the nursing profession for many years to come and did not disappear with the Registration Act of 1919.

In 1900 the Council issued a new agreement for the County Nursing Associations in which it was admitted that the needs of the town and country were different, and that in the country midwifery posed a great challenge. The Council decided that it would sanction the employment of village nurse-midwives where it was impossible to support a Queen's nurse and where the population did not exceed 3000 people, or 'in a district where a Queen's Nurse is already employed and there is a demand for a village nurse for midwifery practice'.

The Council also decreed that Queen's nurses employed by the County Nursing Association should be inspected by, and responsible to, the Queen's Institute Superintendent, while village nurses should be under the supervision of a superintendent of village nurses to be appointed with the assent of the County Nursing Association who would contribute to her salary. Furthermore, village nurses should only live in patients' houses when local circumstances rendered it necessary and such occasions must be reported.[13] At this point Lady Selborne, a supporter of the original Rural District Nursing Association and the formidable daughter of the Marquis of Salisbury, entered the fray. Lady Selborne was the honorary secretary of the Hampshire County Nursing Association, and she believed in local autonomy and regarded with suspicion the rules sent out by the Queen's Institute Council. She objected to there being a separate superintendent for village nurses; she argued that the whole staff should be placed under the control of one county nursing superintendent and subject to inspection by the Institute. Lady Selborne also disagreed about the ruling of village nurses not living in; in her area they did, and they liked it and so did the patients.

The Council discussed Lady Selborne's objections and they agreed that there should be one county nursing superintendent who should have overall surveillance of all district nursing and midwifery in the county, a sensible arrangement that pertained as long as village nurses were employed. On the subject of 'living in' the Council were adamant and the practice died a natural death. This episode is worth recalling not only to trace the historical lineage of the Queen's Institute administrative structure, but to record the social power of some of the county organisations. After all, the Council of the Queen's Institute was appointed by the Queen and it was not easily intimidated. Lady Selborne was not the only formidable honorary secretary to a County Association jealously guarding county autonomy.

As the general nurse training lengthened, the Queen's Institute laid down that village nurses should have at least

One year's training in hospital work;
three months' training in midwifery;
three to six months' training in district work;

and village nurses were trained in other centres at Worcester, Tipton, Leeds, Watford and in Devonshire. This two-tier system of rural district nursing remained in force until the coming of the National Health Service. However, after the Midwives Act of 1936 when

55

midwifery training was lengthened to one year, few village nurses were trained. Nevertheless, during the 50 or so years of their existence village nurses, if properly supervised, played an important part in the raising of the standard of care in the rural community which it was impossible to cover, and would have been extravagant to do so, by Queen's nurses. The purists may fulminate, and legislation may change the legal position of the nurse, but whether she is village nurse, ordinary probationer, or enrolled nurse, it seems that nursing will always need some kind of two-tier system. Either there are not enough highly trained people to undertake all the tasks, or there is not enough money to pay for them, or maybe all tasks do not require highly trained nurses, merely highly trained supervision.

Rural midwives had been a feature of country life from time immemorial. The Bible and Shakespeare are full of references to them, either actual or symbolic. But apart from midwives, the poor, if they could pay, were often assisted by 'handy women'. In 1883 a Miss Broadwood had the idea of organising a Cottage Benefit Nursing Association, which was later known as the Holt–Ockley system after its original locality. By 1909 the scheme, which was run on provident lines from Dennison House in London, was employing some 800 'cottage nurses', of whom about 4 per cent were certified midwives while the rest had little or no training. Miss Broadwood's nurses gave help in the home and they lived in. This, claimed Miss Broadwood, is what the doctors wanted, and as Mary Stocks puts it 'earlier discussions with the BMA suggest that in this particular statement Miss Broadwood spoke nothing but the truth'.[14] While the Queen's Institute accepted village nurses under the supervision of a Queen's Superintendent, they were less happy about a third tier, for they feared, with some justification, that districts might opt for this less expensive service to the detriment of the Institute. However, Miss Broadwood's scheme flourished for some time, providing what was really the prototype of the home help system, and they gave evidence at the Jubilee Congress on District Nursing in 1909.

THE EDWARDIAN PERIOD

The situation at the turn of the century was that there were county nursing associations, some of which were inherited from Mrs Malleson's RDNA, which were now affiliated to the Queen's Institute and subject to the Queen's Inspector. From time to time the affiliation subcommittee varied the conditions, such as agreeing to Queen's superintendents supervising village nurses, and from time to time associations, for one reason or another, disaffiliated. The minutes of the Council are full of persuasion, or reluctant acceptance. Within the counties there were district nursing associations, again some were inherited, and if there was a county nursing association these were affiliated to it, if not, then to the Queen's Institute. These, like the county associations, sometimes fell out of affiliation, either because they broke the rules, or because the Queen's nurse had left and they had substituted an untrained nurse, or because they manifested some sectarian preference. The duties of the County Superintendent were to be responsible to her County Committee for a good standard of nursing work, for interviewing and engaging candidates, for arranging the training and work, for keeping a register and record of all the nurses and their work and for superintending all nurses affiliated to the Association. What is interesting is that within a comparatively short time the Institute had established that nurses were responsible to, and accountable to, nurses for their professional work. Nursing administration had carved itself out an empire, though, as in the hospitals, not without some trauma.

But in spite of the fact that by 1900 there were some 750 Queen's nurses on the Roll with 65 affiliated associations and the Institute was gaining prestige, there were a number of organisations outside. Some, like the Ranyard nurses, had been formed before the Queen's Institute and were precluded from affiliation by their aims and objectives. Others, like the Bristol Nursing Association which had been formed in 1881 on the lines of the Liverpool Association, preferred local autonomy to affiliation which Bristol resisted until 1944.[15] There is an interesting note in the minutes where the Countess of Selborne is deputed to visit the Duchess of Northumberland. Northumberland applied for affiliation and the Duchess asked, if the district was unable to supply a Queen's nurse, could the Council sanction a fully trained hospital nurse on the understanding that after one year's work under inspection, she would be enrolled as a Queen's nurse? This, said the Council firmly, could not be allowed. It is not clear how the Duchess and the Countess resolved the dispute which also centred on the thorny question of the nurse living in, but the minutes record that a grant was eventually made to Northumberland.

It was an uphill struggle. Often the number of disaffiliations equated with the number of affiliations and this may not be unconnected with the fact that although in 1900 nearly 200 names were placed on the Queen's Roll, over 100 Queen's nurses left the service. Why the wastage was so high is not clear, but one reason was probably economic. The local associations paid the salary of the nurse, and often this compared unfavourably with salaries offered elsewhere. Another reason was that in a period of late marriage the marriage rate of these eminently eligible nurses was high. Moreover, the work was physically hard and a strain on the health of young nurses and, sadly, many left for health reasons.

Part of the problem stemmed from the lack of finance and the uncertain way in which it was collected at local level. Given a good donation the Association could afford a Queen's nurse, given a bad year it could not. Although the Queen's Commemorative Fund had brought a further £84 000 to the Institute, the income on this did little to provide for the growing needs of the service. Appeals for new money were on the whole disappointing and this was partly due to the changing ethos and social philosophy.

When the Queen's Institute was founded, the only refuge for the sick poor was the outpatient department of a charity hospital or the Poor Law. The prevailing philosophy of social Darwinism was that the fit and the worthy would survive by their own efforts and self-help. Now with the great depression of the mid–1870s to the 1890s, the high unemployment that was to figure in Booth's survey, and the humiliations of the Boer War and its sad record of the health of recruits, people were beginning to question the assumption that health could be left to charity and that poverty could be avoided by thrift. As the industrial revolution ran out of steam and competition increased, some people began to have doubts about the whole economic system. There was the rise of trade unionism, especially in the skilled trades, and the emergence of the Labour Party with its various strands. The new breed of social scientists like Charles Booth, Seebohm Rowntree and the Webbs began to argue in favour of state insurance and government intervention. The rise of municipal authorities after the Local Government Act 1888 meant that they now assumed, albeit sometimes haphazardly, control of some public health services. If some, why not others?

Above all, the old Victorian caste society was breaking up. Values, taboos and social habits were in the melting pot. The King, 'the most exalted person in the land was seen playing cards for money and had answered disagreeable questions in the divorce courts.'[16] The social mores were changing. Lady Georgina, distributing wine and rabbits to grateful cottagers expecting nothing but deference, was becoming a thing of the past. In spite of its portrayal as a Golden Age before the storm of the First World War, the Edwardian period was fraught with social unrest. The falling prices in the latter part of the nineteenth century meant that in spite of low wages the standard of living for those in work had risen; this was now reversed, prices rose, the standard of living fell, and there was much poverty. This meant there were great demands on the Queen's nurses. People were ill because they were poor and poor because they were ill, and it also meant that there was less chance of getting donations from patients.

George Cole has described the Edwardian period as being like the first two acts of a play in which the third was never written.[16] The various movements of revolt and the tentative measures for reform were brought to an abrupt halt in early August 1914. Some measures, like the Education Act of 1918, were picked up again when the war was over, but many reforms like the intended reform of the health services were postponed because of interwar unemployment and the economic crisis. In many cases they had to wait for another war before those measures could be tackled again and the third act could be written. The Queen's nurses, founded as a Victorian charity, had to weather these vicissitudes as best they could. That they spearheaded a universal community nursing service of high quality is a testimony to the ingenuity of the Council in making ends meet, and the esteem in which the Queen's nurses were held.

NOTES

1. Clark, W. *Thoughts on the Management and Relief of the Poor*, Bath Tracts, 1825 Bath Reference Library.
2. Alexander, C.M. *Hymns Ancient and Modern* no. 573, 1848.
3. Fraser, D. *The Evolution of the British Welfare State*, Macmillan, London, 1973, p. 115.
4. Shaw, G.B. *Major Barbara*, Odhams Press, London, 1905, Act 2.
5. Maggs, C.J. *Origins of General Nursing*, Croom Helm, London, 1983, p. 43.
6. Hanbury Parochial Nurse's Diary 1869–1875, compiled by Lady Georgina Vernon, QIN.
7. Baly, M.E. *Florence Nightingale and the Nursing Legacy*, Croom Helm, London, 1986, Chapter 5.
8. Malleson, H. *The Life of Elizabeth Malleson of Dixton Manor* 1828–1916, privately printed 1926.
9. Donnison, J. *Midwives and Medical Men*, Heinemann, London, 1977.
10. Abel-Smith, B. *A History of the Nursing Profession*, Heinemann, London, 1960, p. 5.
11. W. Rathbone/ P. Peter 11 May 1896, QNI.
12. Baly, M.E. *Florence Nightingale and the Nursing Legacy*, Croom Helm, London, 1986, pp. 206–7.
13. Council Minutes, 17 October 1900, QNI.

14. Stocks, M. *A Hundred Years of District Nursing*, Allen and Unwin, London, 1960, p. 134.

15. Inspector's Report, PRO 60/63 113, 1944.

16. Cole, G.D.H. and Postgate, R. *The Common People*, Methuen, London, 1968, pp. 452–3.

5

The Queen's Nurses at the Beginning of the Century

Queen Victoria died in 1901 and her place as patron of the Institute was taken by Queen Alexandra, who already had an interest in nursing. The founders of the Institute were disappearing. William Rathbone, the wise father figure, had died at the age of 83 years in 1902, and had been succeeded at the Institute by his son, William Gair Rathbone. The Duke of Westminster, who had been associated with district nursing since the founding of the Metropolitan and National Nursing Association, had lived to perform his last task, the winding up of the Commemoration Fund, and Florence Nightingale, now over 80 years old, had ceased to play an active part in nursing matters. However, her vision of the district nurse as an educated health missionary, was carried on by disciples like Mrs Craven, Rosalind Paget and Amy Hughes.

THE INSTITUTE COUNCIL

By the end of the first decade of the century the Council of the Queen's Institute had grown to 68 members. The President was the Duke of Devonshire and the trustees were the Duke of Norfolk, the Duke of Portland and Lord Rothschild, while the Council itself had three royal princesses and a posse of countesses and duchesses usually representing the County Nursing Associations. However, the main work was done on committees with two members of the Rathbone family, William Gair and Rosalind Paget; two members of the Bonham Carter family, Henry and Maurice; with other longstanding stalwarts like Sir Dyce Duckworth, of the Royal College of Physicians, the Reverend Dacre Craven, Harold Boulton and Mrs Minet. It is interesting that no less than seven of the working members were also members of the Nightingale Fund Council, were associated with St Thomas's Hospital, and were well versed in new ideas on nurse training.

Meetings of the Institute Council continued to be held at St Katherine's Hospital under the Presidency of the Master, the Reverend Arthur Peile, but the minutes indicate that the relationship was not always happy, the promised benefaction was not forthcoming, and the Institute gained little from the marriage. The work of the Institute was growing and it needed accommodation that was more central. In 1902 the Council set up a subcommittee to consider the relationship of the Institute with St Katherine's.[1] The report, presented to Queen Alexandra, asked yet again if there were any prospect of money from St Katherine's, and in a letter the Council ventured to suggest that it was 'not in the long-term interest for the Master of St Katherine's to be the President of the Institute since future Masters may have neither the inclination nor the aptitude for the work connected with the Institute'. The Queen accepted that in future the Master of St Katherine's should not necessarily be the President of the Institute, but on the subject of financial aid from the funds of St Katherine's the Queen could promise nothing. It is not clear why the refusal was so adamant. There was no evidence that the Order was reforming its activities after the criticism by the Lord Chancellor, and the Order was dissolved in 1914.[2]

In June the following statement was presented by the Master to the Council:

Her Majesty having had various matters brought before her notice with reference to the relations which at present exist between St Katherine's Royal Hospital and the Queen's Institute for Nurses has come to the conclusion that it is to the interest of both that the connexion between them should cease and that the Institute should provide rooms and offices for the Queen's Nurses' staff elsewhere. In order to facilitate such arrangements Her Majesty has been graciously pleased to give £1,000 so that the expenses necessarily incident to such a change may not burden the Institute.[3]

This gift enabled the Queen's Institute to establish an independent home of its own in 120 Victoria Street and it marks the beginning of a new phase.

THE INSTITUTE AND THE COLONIES

Meanwhile the work of the Institute had spread to the Empire. Lady Aberdeen, the wife of the Governor of Canada from 1893 to 1897, conceived the idea of starting a Queen Victoria Order of district nurses in Canada on the lines of the Queen's Institute in the United Kingdom, and in a letter to the Duke of Westminster she claimed that the Queen had given permission for the badge of the Institute to be given to nurses in Canada. An order had been given to Bent and Parker for their badges to be despatched, and they in turn had written to the Queen Victoria's Jubilee Institute for samples of ribbon and cord. This was the first the Council had heard of the matter and the President, the Reverend Peile, was perhaps justifiably indignant. Badges should only be given to nurses who were in an Association affiliated to the Queen's Institute and who were duly inspected by the Queen's inspector, and he wrote accordingly: 'Canada cannot have the badge because it is not affiliated to the Institute. The Council should be consulted before permission is given . . . .'.[4]

There followed a series of urgent cables because Lady Aberdeen was anxious to launch her scheme before she left Canada. In vain she pleaded. Peile at last conceded that there would be no objection to the use of the badge, but he objected to the use of the brassard, the ribbon and the cord, and he suggested that it would be better if the badge were suspended by a ribbon of different colour. The incident, involving, as it did, the top echelons of the aristocracy, serves to indicate how quickly the honour of being a Queen's nurse had impressed itself. The whole episode, however, belies the picture of the Reverend Peile as being a mere figurehead; he had grasped the principle at stake perhaps better than some of his Council. In a letter to the Duke of Westminster he wrote:

The more I think of it the less it commends itself that which is a distinguishing mark of the Queen's Nurses in the United Kingdom should be the same in Canada. We cannot have any control as to the training of Canadian nurses and as we each have a separate charter we had better be entirely independent in all respects.[5]

In the end Lady Aberdeen got her badges and ribbons though she agreed to a different uniform. Peile wrote one last despairing letter to the Duke and accepted the *fait accompli*.

The point raised by Peile was not academic and it was soon to be raised in a wider issue. Pride in the Empire and the Diamond Jubilee celebrations led to a spate of requests from the colonies and a difference of opinion as to how these requests should be accommodated. Walter Hely-Hutchinson, the Governor General of Cape Town, South Africa, had established a Victoria Nurses' Institute as a Jubilee Commemoration, and he then appealed for federation with England, pointing out that, alas, because of the Boer War the Institute had no money. The Council of the Institute considered the request, but decided that the system operating in South Africa, where nurses were provided for private nursing and not for the sick poor, did not meet with the Institute's rules.[6] A request from Tasmania for affiliation was turned down for the same reason.

However, Harold Boulton, now Honorary Secretary to the Institute, was an advocate for a wider role and he and fellow Council members drew up proposals for the Federation of Colonial Nursing Associations to the Queen Victoria Jubilee Institute. The proposals set forth the advantages of Federation: 'mutual help and support, the raising of the standard of training and the services to the Sick Poor by thoroughly trained nurses'. Conditions for affiliation were to be much the same as those laid down for associations affiliated to the Institute in the United Kingdom and would include inspection of work to be made regularly by trained officers. It was further proposed that: 'Two or three Colonial Inspectors in London should be constantly travelling to help in organising local associations in the colonies and to advise and inspect those already established . . . '.[7]

In the end no such formal organisation was set up, presumably because the Institute had neither the money nor the personnel for such a venture; by the time it had, the sun had set on the British Empire and a less formal contact was required. Nevertheless, the prestige of the Queen's Institute had spread abroad. A Miss Kruysee from Holland had been to England for training under Miss Dunn and had returned to set up a district nursing service in Amsterdam. In Sweden a Miss Lind ap Hagely procured papers from England and set about organising the work there, and, as the Congress in Liverpool in 1909 showed, there had been an exchange of information between other countries, some of whom had adopted Queen's methods to suit their own needs. South Australia had had a district nursing service since 1894, and when they were anxious to make improvement the Institute allowed its General Superintendent, Miss Amy Hughes, to go to Australia for six months to help organise a scheme on the lines of the Queen's Institute. Hereafter a number of Queen's nurses were to act as advisers to countries who wished to start a system of district nurse training, but in each case the scheme had to be adapted to meet the peculiar needs of different countries.

DEVELOPMENT OF THE INSTITUTE IN THE UNITED KINGDOM

Meanwhile in the United Kingdom the work of the Institute progressed. Inspectors were sent out to draw up agreements with affiliated associations on the lines laid down by the Institute and then to inspect the work of the Queen's nurses employed. One recurring difficulty was finance. How was the money to be raised by the local association to pay for the nurse? The inspector on several occasions had to write:

> The Council of the Queen's Institute, while approving the encouragement of contributions from patients, whether voluntary or by fixed charges on the provident system, strongly disapproves of charges for the nurse's services being made by the visit or the nurse being responsible for the collection of fees . . .[8]

By the first years of the twentieth century the Council had come round to the view that the Associations should give consideration to raising money by organising provident schemes, and model rules were sent out, stressing always that services to necessitous cases should be free. In 1910 Amy Hughes gave a paper to the Charity Organisation Society,[9] in which she set out suggested guidelines for collecting money on the basis of the weekly income of wage-earners in the district. Such exhortations to thrift and the preparation for a rainy day fitted well with the philosophy of the Charity Organisation Society, who were currently arguing against the need for government intervention and state insurance. However, it is not clear how many associations availed themselves of this method; collection of dues was difficult and time-consuming. The Queen's Institute was now facing the problem that was engaging the government: how to provide for the troughs of adversity among the poor, so well described by Booth. Could this be done by voluntary effort? Or was there a need for government action?

Rural life in golden Edwardian England was not always salubrious. An inspector's report for 1906 tells of

> Ten cases of typhoid and one death in a row of cottages where the rooms were without windows and fireplaces and the only water supply from a stream at the side of the road, that was nearly dried

up. . . . The nurses were dealing with typhoid cases night and day . . .[10]

Not surprisingly, one nurse had 'broken down'. Not only were district nurses nursing epidemics of typhoid, which, of course, hospitals would not accept, they were tackling a wide range of medical and surgical nursing. What was expected of district nurses at that time can be gathered from the advice given in *Nursing Notes*, and after 1904 in the *Queen's Nurses' Magazine* and the examination papers of the times. That the nurses were expected to prepare the patient and the room for surgical operations in homes and be the doctor's assistant is clear from the detailed advice given about sweeping chimneys, disinfecting dustbins, getting rid of pets and preparing the kitchen table for the operation. After the operation the nurse is exhorted to restore the patient with: 'smelling salts, 3 pennyworth of brandy, a fan, ice, strong coffee and a new laid egg'.[11] Operations in the home were commonplace because not all areas were served with hospitals. There were many cases hospitals would not accept, and 'home operation saved the disruption of the family' and, many argued, not without some justification, home was safer. Extracts from nurses' reports show the wide range of operations being undertaken:

I have not had any big operations lately. Some of them were: Amputation of leg (close to hip joint) ventral hernia, appendicitis with perforation, inguinal hernia and haemorrhoids. Of course I have had a lot of small ones . . .

and

. . . I get a variety of operations, ovariotomy (several) Lithotrity, Extra Uterine, Herniotomy, Caesarean Section, Amputation of Breast, fingers, toes (but no legs) glands, cysts, tracheotomy, and of course tonsils, adenoids and circumcisions any amount also several nephrotomies, appendicitis . . .[12]

Apart from showing surgical skills and ingenuity of a high order and wrestling with infections, fever epidemics and dealing with the many medical diseases that afflicted the poor, the Queen's nurse was a school nurse, health educator, and now, with more emphasis being placed on infant care, the adviser to mothers and families on infant welfare. How much maternity work was undertaken by the Queen's nurses is uncertain. It would seem that most districts employed special maternity nurses or midwives; it was considered uneconomic for

Queen's nurses to take maternity cases because of the uncertainty of the time factor and because of the risk of infection. However, by the time of the Liverpool Congress in 1909, speakers were urging the district nurse to extend her duties to antenatal care, and, in rural areas, to embrace the whole gamut of maternal care and education. To add to her multifarious duties she was now urged to give lectures to adolescent girls on the subject of motherhood.[13] Small wonder that some lecturers at the Congress asked if 'they had come to the parting of the ways', and that more than one type of nurse or health worker was needed in the community.

Earlier there are descriptions of Queen's nurses dealing with childbirth in bizarre situations. An article in *Nursing Notes* for 1898 shows that life was full of incident. On Christmas night the nurse was called away from dealing with a pleurisy case to a man who had had a fall from a horse which rolled on him 'injuring him most terribly'. Here she was summoned by a girl of ten years to say the 'mother was bad' and was led to a caravan at the bottom of Muddy Lane where she climbed over the shafts to find mother in labour on the floor with husband and seven children around her. There was no room to undress the mother so she was delivered on her knees on the floor and eventually put her on the bed with three other children and the baby with three more children in boxes under the bed. Lady Lambton who recorded the story spoke warmly of the nurse's ingenuity and the parents' gratitude saying: 'The Queen would be pleased that one of her nurses attended a gipsy mother on Christmas night in a van down Muddy Lane carrying out Her Majesty's thoughtful care for her poorer subjects'.[14] Lady Lambton was a member of the Council of the Institute, and she herself paid a visit to the van down Muddy Lane, presumably climbing over the shafts. Like Mr Rathbone, she knew about the work of district nurses first hand.

INSPECTION AND EXAMINATIONS

One of the innovations of the time was the periodic inspection of the nurse's work by the inspector sent from headquarters. The reports reveal that the Institute was concerned with the nurse as a whole person and as an example to her neighbourhood. There was no distinction between on duty and off duty. In Boxford it was recorded:

> work excellent, very neat capable nurse. Baskets beautifully neat and well fitted. Books in order. Nurse shares house with friend

who sometimes takes a private case. They have no maid. (*sic*) Everything about the house and all the details most finished and neat . . .

But, alas, in the next district: 'Books not well kept, lives alone, house untidy. Is liked by patients . . . is inclined to give a great deal of time to some and to neglect others. I have advised Miss Perceval not to keep her'.[15]

In report after report the main concern was that the nurse should be neat, orderly and tactful and her whole life an inspiration to orderly habits in the neighbourhood. It was in the Nightingale tradition. Miss Nightingale once wrote: 'ward training is but half training. The other half consists in women being trained in habits of order, cleanliness, regularity and moral discipline [in the Nurses' Home]'. Nurses' cottages or rooms, like baskets and books, were open to the strictest inspection.

The rift with Liverpool

The progress to inspection and written examinations with the district nurses being given more responsibility was not universally smooth. Liverpool, which had started a system of district nursing based on Ladies' Committees, with nurses accountable to a Lady Superintendent had never happily accepted the London domination of the Queen's Institute. Now, in 1907, it objected to the examinations that were being imposed on the candidates for the Queen's Roll. Mrs Rathbone wrote a series of pungent letters pointing out that potentially good nurses were frightened by examinations: 'Are these unliterary but skilled women to be rejected in favour of good talkers and writers . . . '[16]

This was an argument that was to continue for many a year and did not cease with Mrs Rathbone. Liverpool flatly refused to carry out the Institute's scheme of theoretical lectures and examinations and they persuaded some of their northern colleagues to do likewise. This led to a rift in the Rathbone family with a long, well-reasoned letter by Rosalind Paget putting the case for the Institute. The letter is interesting because it has a modern ring setting out the argument that good nursing and intelligent understanding of theory are not mutually exclusive and that modern developments in sanitary science meant that more was required of, and expected of, the nurse. Miss Paget said that in her considerable experience of examining nurses she found that those who failed examinations or were deferred often had a poor nursing report. Miss Paget dealt with the criticisms of the examination paper for 1909 which show that the candidates were expected to have some knowledge of health legislation, of school nursing and its legislation, appropriate advice to adolescents, the teaching of hygiene and the preparation for an operation in the home. The district nurse was meant to be a health visitor to all age groups and the provider of medical and surgical skills in the home. This was not Liverpool's concept of district nursing; health teaching was, in their opinion, best left to the lay committee. Miss Paget's views were endorsed by the Council of the Institute who endeavoured to pour oil on troubled water, but the dispute rankled for some time and it had not subsided when Liverpool decided to hold a Jubilee Congress to mark its 50 years of district nursing.

The Jubilee Congress

The Report and Proceedings of the Jubilee Congress give a kaleidoscopic picture of district nursing in the first decade of the century. By no means all the organisations represented were affiliated to the Queen's Institute. In fact it would seem that Liverpool wanted to emphasise that the Queen's Institute was only one among many, a comparative newcomer, and there was an undercurrent of rivalry and a certain amount of animosity. Rosalind Paget, in a letter to her cousin Willie Rathbone, expressed doubts about Liverpool's loyalty to the wider cause:

> I can't help feeling that some of them [the Liverpool Association] are inclined to emphasise the work your father did in starting District Work in Liverpool rather than bring forward the work he did in creating the Queen Victoria Institute which was for *everywhere* . . . the spirit of antagonism to the Q.V.I. by all the Liverpool people has lately been so obvious that one can't ignore it — they seem set against all development and going forward. Now the question of your father's many qualities was his power of development — he was young to the last days of his life.[17]

Nevertheless, the Congress was a remarkable achievement. Delegates came from Holland, Sweden, Germany, Norway, Australia, Bulgaria, France, and the United States, and all gave papers on the organisation of district nursing in their countries. Many, however, would not have passed the affiliation test of the Queen's Institute, some were religious organisations and were definitely sectarian; not all employed trained nurses and a number combined private work with district work. With the exception of Canada, none was modelled on the Queen's Institute.

Apart from papers from different countries, there were lectures on different aspects of district nursing ranging through the psychological aspect of nursing, the prevention of tuberculosis, maternity nursing, school nursing to pensions and salaries. The lecture on pensions casts an interesting light on the life of district nurses at that time. It was argued that district nurses could not make provision for their retirement, not, as one would have thought, because their salaries were so low, but because:

> three or four years of training are required, it results, therefore, that a woman is 27 or 28 before she is qualified to work on her own account — if she wants to do so; before she can earn anything but the most trifling sum together with her board and lodging . . . the age at which a nurse must cease to work is not absolute but experience of this and similar institutions shows that some nurses begin to find difficulty in obtaining work after the age of 40, that most nurses have difficulty in obtaining employment after the age of 45 and very few can earn a livelihood at 50 years.[18]

Mr Dick, the secretary of the Royal National Pension Fund for Nurses, mentions the new government old age pension, but that only applied to people aged 70, and there was therefore, a 20-year gap. These rather startling figures are borne out by the statistics of the Queen's Institute. In 1909, after 20 years of existence, the Institute had 1665 Queen's nurses. That year they enrolled 281, but in 1910 the figure had only risen to 1795, which means that 149 nurses on the Roll had left, and the same pattern can be traced throughout the decade. At least 100 leave the service each year, and among the reasons for leaving the most prominent are marriage, private nursing and 'on account of health' and, of course, many who went into private nursing probably did so for reasons of health. The district nurse's life was hard and some died in the course of duty, often from infection contracted during their visits to homes and schools.

NEW DEMANDS FOR HEALTH CARE

One thing was clear from the Congress papers, that the new demands for health care were pressing heavily on this small service. Nurses were urged to run clinics for mothers and babies, to visit schools, to encourage thrift, to supervise rehabilitation, to undertake maternity cases and to be ready at any time to assist with the appendectomy on the kitchen table. Was the role too wide and could one training encompass it all? Already the split into specialities was beginning to occur. The new London County Council in 1904 started to employ a separate group of nurses, who were not district nurses, to manage the health of school children in London and to be responsible to the Medical Officers of Health.

Other cities, seeing the advantage of this system, and responding to new legislation, followed suit giving rise to the autonomous system of school nursing that characterised many cities in the twentieth century. Since the end of the nineteenth century some local authorities had employed women as health visitors to carry the sanitary message to the poor. In 1892 Buckinghamshire provided a special training and now, in 1908, a special course was provided by Bedford College. Some authorities, pressed again by legislation, had begun to employ a definite corps of health visitors, some of whom had a nurse training, some had not. The health visitors were giving advice and guidance and intervening in child welfare which the district nurse saw as their duty. Examination questions show that district nurses were expected to know about the safeguards for fostering children under the 1908 Act. However, there is no suggestion from district nurses themselves, or from their very articulate leaders, that they saw the necessity to give up part of their function to another group. Nevertheless, they were nurses first, and one gets the impression that they saw the physical needs of the necessitous poor as their first priority, and the inspector's reports continue to concentrate on the neatness of baskets, the order of books and cupboards, the correctness of uniform and the relationship with the sick patient.

NOTES

1. Queen's Institute of Nursing Minutes, 8 October 1902
2. Jamison, C. *History of the Royal Hospital of St Katherine's*, Oxford University Press, Oxford, 1952.
3. Stocks, M. *A Hundred Years of District Nursing*, Allen and Unwin,

London, 1960, p. 117.

4. A. Peile/Lady Aberdeen 8 September 1898.

5. A. Peile/Duke of Westminster 21 October 1899.

6. H. Boulton/W. Hely-Hutchinson undated 1901.

7. Note on colonial branches attributed to W. Rathbone, 1910.

8. Inspector's report, Berkshire 1905, PRO 20/63/4.

9. Hughes, A. *District Nursing on Provident Lines*, Reprinted Charity Organisation Society, 1910.

10. Inspector's report, Wantage 1906, PRO 30/63/4.

11. *Nursing Notes*, Vol. XI February 1898, article M.J. Loane.

12. Extracts from letters from Queen's nurses, October 1909, Queen's Institute.

13. Report and Proceedings of the Liverpool Congress, Marples and Co. Liverpool, 1909, p. 145f.

14. *Nursing Notes*, February 1898. How a Queen's nurse spent Christmas Night, by Victoria Lambton.

15. Inspector's report, Boxford 1905, PRO 30/63/4.

16. E. Rathbone/Miss Gillie 2 October 1909, Picton Library, Liverpool.

17. R. Paget/W.G. Rathbone, quoted Mary Stocks, p. 127, undated.

18. Report of the Liverpool Congress: Pensions for Nurses, pp. 280–1.

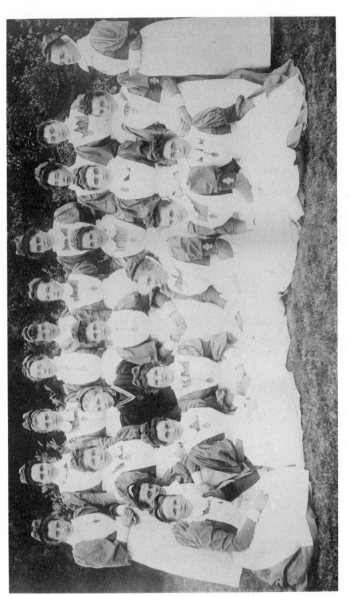

Plate 1. Queen's Nurses at the Turn of the Century.

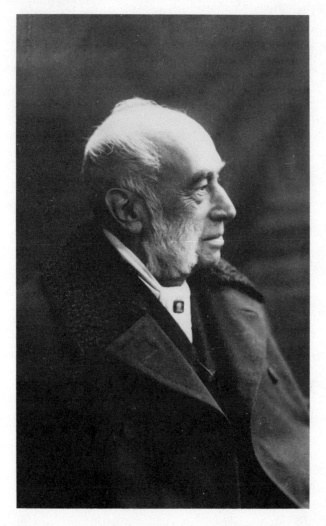

Plate 2. William Rathbone (1819-1902) Founder of
District Nursing, Liverpool, 1859.

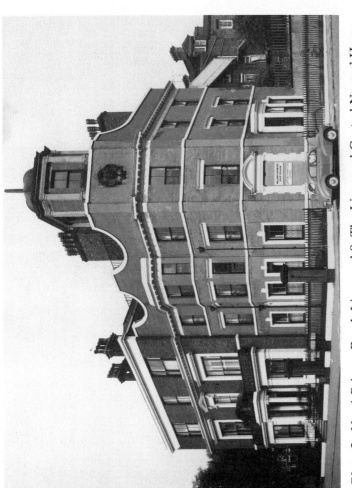

Plate 3. No. 1 Princes Road, Liverpool 8. The Liverpool Central Nurses' Home and later the William Rathbone Staff College.

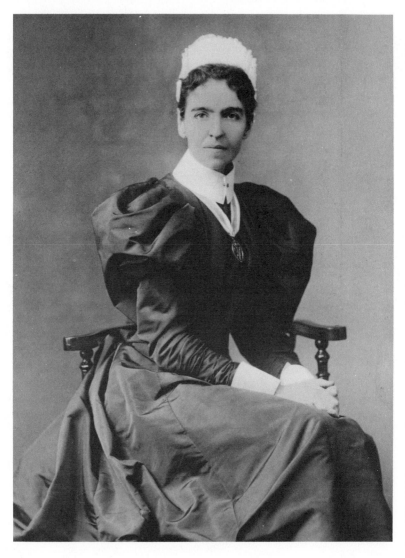

Plate 4. Dame Rosalind Paget, 1st Queen's Nurse and Inspector, 1890-1891.

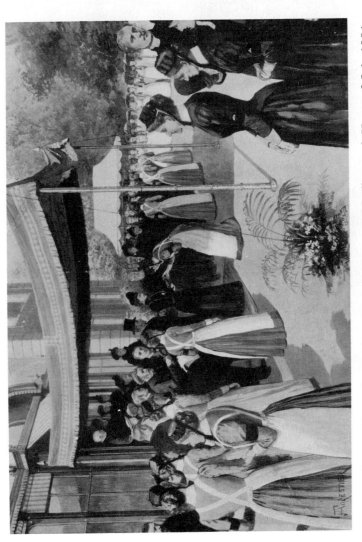

Plate 5. Queen Alexandra receives Queen's Nurses at Marlborough House, 3 July 1901.

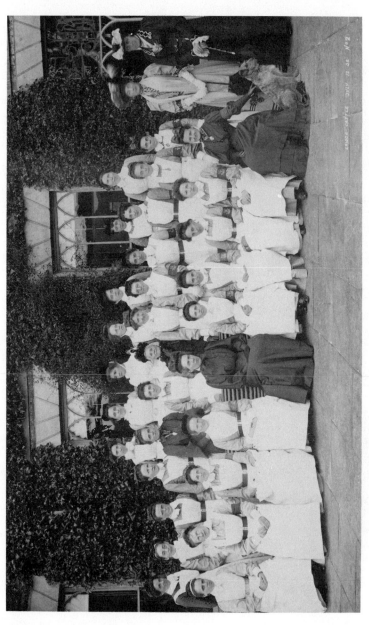

Plate 6. Sussex County Nursing Association, Eridge Castle, 12 July 1906.

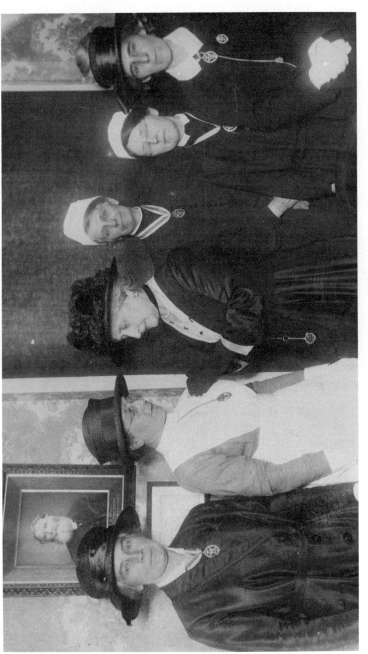

Plate 7. Presentation of the 'Gold Medal'. 21 years' Service with the Institute, 1910.

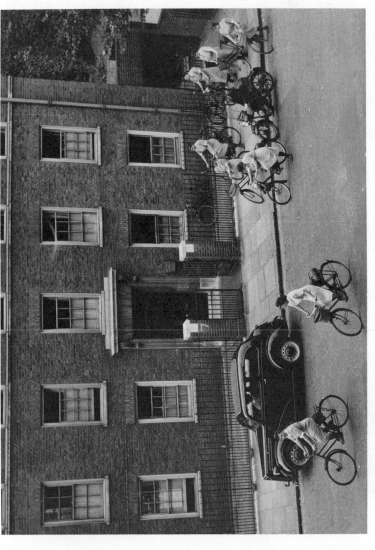

Plate 8. Working from a Home. Queen's Nurses Begin their Daily Rounds.

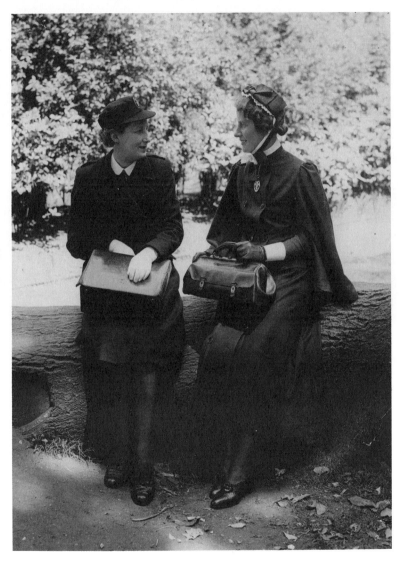

Plate 9. Uniform (*c*. 1925 and *c*. 1950).

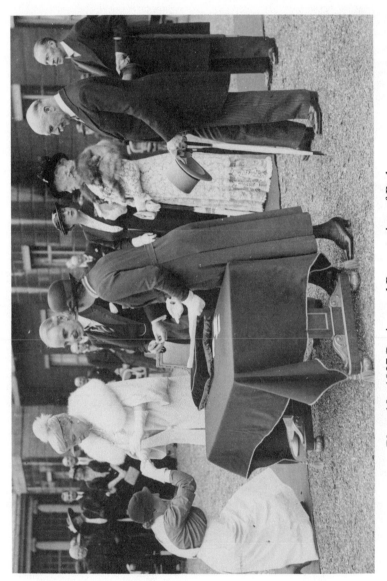

Plate 10. 1937 Review and Presentation of Badges.

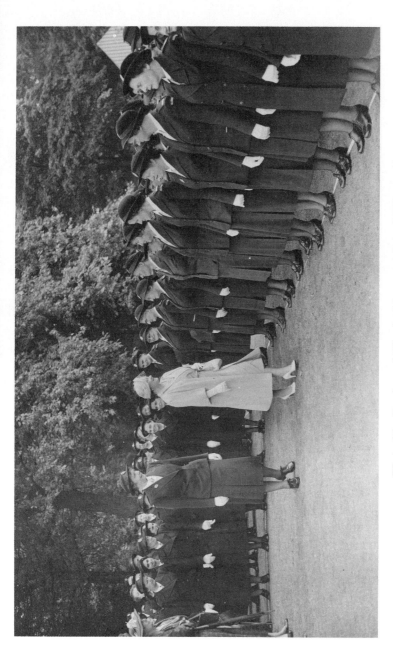

Plate 11. Review of District Nurses, 1 July 1959.

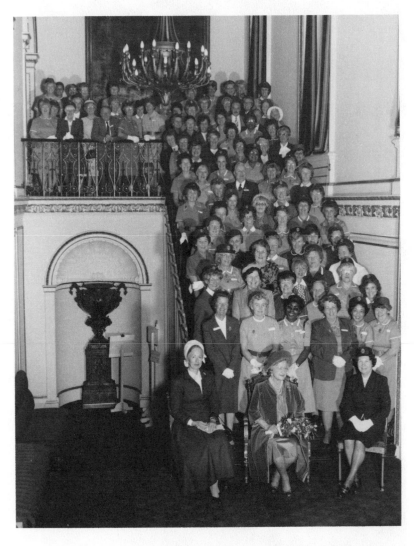

Plate 12. The Long Service Badge Ceremony at St James's
Palace, 20 November 1985.

6

District Nursing: Charity or Public Service?

At the beginning of the century, apart from charity, the main source of help to the necessitous poor was relief from the Poor Law, but this had become anachronistic. Amended in 1834 on the mistaken concept that it was the immobile, able-bodied poor who were putting up the rates, the new law had endeavoured to force mobility and employment by the principle of less eligibility. All too soon it was found that workhouses were full of the old, children, the disabled and the sick. Reform movements abounded and piecemeal attempts had been made to deal with the problem. Workhouse infirmaries had been built, and the principle of less eligibility had become less rigid; nevertheless, it was generally admitted that the law was chaotic and was trying to accommodate two systems with opposing aims: deterrence and welfare.

In 1905 Balfour, in virtually his last act as Prime Minister, set up a Royal Commission on the Poor Law, but the report did not appear until 1909. The commissioners included leading churchmen, members of the Charity Organisation Society with whom the Queen's Institute had contact, Octavia Hill, and social workers like Charles Booth and Beatrice Webb. The Commissioners, who heard a mass of evidence, were clearly troubled about the obsolete state of the law especially as it related to the sick poor, and the majority of the members, led by Octavia Hill, defended the principle of less eligibility as a spur to work, and they feared that state provision would lead to a falling off of voluntary subscriptions and undermine the whole concept of charity.

Octavia Hill, like the writers to *The Times*, saw the provision of school meals as a menace to the incentive of working class mothers. On the other hand, Mrs Webb, a Fabian socialist, disagreed and wrote her own minority report which proposed the break up of the Poor

Law and, under local authorities, the institution of a complete public health service without any taint of pauperism. One interesting recommendation in Mrs Webb's report was that the local health authority should exercise control over all preventive and curative health services and that they should operate from health centres.[1] Although Mrs Webb's report was one of the inspirations for the National Health Service, curative and preventive services were not brought under one authority until 1974. Apart from its unacceptability to the powerful charity lobby, Mrs Webb's report was damned by the medical profession. It proposed that doctors should be paid a salary.

The Queen's Institute followed these reports with anxiety. Wedded to the voluntary principle, they were disciples of Octavia Hill. What they wanted was the *status quo*, but with increased payments to the district associations for the work they did on behalf of the poor. At the Liverpool Congress, the year of the commission's report, Mr D.F. Pennant, now Honorary Secretary to the Queen's Institute, reminded his audience that of the £108 000 spent on providing Queen's nurses in England and Wales, the Boards of Guardians contributed only 3½ per cent.[2] The Institute now pressed for an increase but to little avail. In a time of social unrest local authorities were sensitive to the issue of rates, and in towns at least they were often training their own nurses.

REFORMING LEGISLATION

Other reforming legislation by the incoming Liberal government was watched with interest by the Institute. Apart from the controversial school meals provision, there was the Education Act of 1907 which set out to provide medical inspection and care for school children. Queen's nurses had been acting as school nurses in many areas since the 1890s and examination papers showed that the Institute considered this as part of their duties. Now, however, these services were put under the authority of the Medical Officer of Health, who sometimes preferred to use health visitors who were accountable to him. On the other hand, when the Institute pressed for payment for the work they did in schools, some authorities, like the London County Council, responded by employing their own school nurses and making them responsible to the local authority. In many areas the Queen's nurse was being squeezed out of her role as a school nurse.

The other piece of legislation to affect the Institute was the National Insurance Act of 1911. The Chancellor of the Exchequer, David Lloyd George, had been to Germany to study the insurance system there where Bismarck had headed off the threat of socialism by a system of benefits paid for by contributions. Back in England Lloyd George set about applying the system there, and although it fell short of its original conception it was a triumph of compromise. It provided for manual workers to make a contribution of 4d a week to an approved society, the employers to pay 3d and the state to pay 2d. It entitled the worker, though not his dependants, to a free choice of doctor from those whose names were on a 'panel' organised by the insurance commissioners. The insurance aspect of the scheme gave it a certain respectability and therefore the approval of the Queen's Institute. That the poor workers could call on medical aid was helpful because the nurse's work was often hampered because the poor could not afford a doctor. However, as the records and anecdotal material show, comparatively few of the district nurse's patients came into the category of insured work. All too often the patients were the old, the children, the disabled and the chronically sick, or wornout mothers.

The National Insurance Act was originally opposed by the doctors because they feared 'panel practice', but at a conference in 1912[3] Mr Pennant said that district nurses should support the Act and that 'the provision of a visiting nurse should be an essential part of the scheme'. He regretted that because of unemployment and mobility of labour it had not been possible to establish a thorough provident system for the payment of district nurses, but now, under Section 21 of the Act, approved societies were allowed to make donations for the support of district nurses visiting and nursing the insured sick, and Mr Pennant suggested that these might take over organising such a system for district nursing: 'I do not suggest that you do away with the charitable part of the work, because you would throw the whole thing into the hands of the State, which most of us think would be undesirable.'

The Institute wanted to be faithful to its foundation and to preserve its voluntary and independent status, but to be subsidised by the State for the services it provided to the insured population. This is what happened, although often on a very unsatisfactory basis. The Act was never implemented as intended, leaving a legacy of confusion after the First World War only to be sorted out by the Beveridge plan in the Second World War.

EDWARDIAN LIFE AND MISS LOANE

Meanwhile, the Queen's nurses, financed in a variety of ways, went about their multifarious duties in town and country wherever an affiliated Association operated. Probably the best insight into the Queen's nurses in the Edwardian period and their attitudes to the social problems of the day is to be found in the writings of the leaders in their journals and published books. Miss Loane, a Queen's Superintendent, published a number of books which were, in their day, bestsellers and popular with the general public; they are lively narrative accounts of the trials of district nurses containing delightful cameo portraits of what she calls the 'respectable poor' whose cause she was championing. *The Daily Chronicle* wrote of one book:

> Miss Loane's information is fresh and direct, and she never fails to be interesting. She could not be dull if she were to try, and although she gives us successive books on social problems, viewed humanly, she does not repeat herself.[4]

Miss Loane was clearly on the side of the majority report on the Poor Law and she, and other leaders of the Queen's nurses, were imbued with the ideas of the Eugenics Movement which, in fact, advertised its meetings in the *Queen's Nurses' Magazine*. Miss Loane was well educated, what Miss Nightingale would have described as a 'superior person', and she quietly lets us know that her patients saw her as such and she, with her nurses, were thus able to educate them. She does not deprecate the poverty of the labouring classes, or their sometimes appalling housing, but she sees them as a challenge to thrift, perseverance, discipline and self-improvement. In a revealing chapter on state spread tables[5] Miss Loane inveighs against school meals and she argues:

> if the State undertook to provide dinners for school children ignorant mothers would be left in the same, or increasing state of ignorance, lazy mothers would become yet more idle; the extravagance of Saturday and Sunday meals would be increased. . . . Industrious mothers, set free from cooking for their children, would seek paid employment . . . this would lower wages for widows and spinsters and ultimately lower wages for men.

Another argument against school meals is set out in her book *The Next Street But One* and has a contemporary ring: 'would not the overworked school teacher rebel at serving meals'.

Miss Loane and her fellow superintendents had their own remedies against the poor feeding of children. Those who cannot feed their children properly should not have them, though Miss Loane, who is a Roman Catholic, does not expound how this is to be achieved, and she has some interesting things to say about taking children into care and using removal as a threat. It is all in the spirit of eugenics, the breeding of a fitter race from the best. And how were parents to be made better? All girls were to be taught cooking at school, and those who were not in domestic service should be compelled to attend classes in cooking, nursing and the care of children. Parish magazines should cut out the sentimental twaddle and devote sections to hygiene and housekeeping, and free leaflets should be distributed. In fact, everything should be done to make the respectable poor more respectable and, of course, content with their lot, though Miss Loane does suggest that working-class mothers should rebel against their small cooking ovens.

The books are full of anecdotes about the poor managing large families in the face of adversity, and by hard work and prudence (and possibly a small allotment) somehow making ends meet, of course, duly guided and advised by the district nurse and the lady superintendent. Today, it all sounds slightly patronising, but Miss Loane's books reflect the social attitudes of the times and the firm conviction that the 'worthy poor' with guidance could be improved *within* the social order, a conviction that the coming war, with its shared sacrifice, was to dent, if not shatter. It is interesting that Miss Loane, who obviously loves her clients, declares she has seldom met real poverty, by which she means absolute destitution, and she seems to have little patience with unemployment, assuming that all who seek long enough will find work. However, in spite of this somewhat rosy view of the labouring poor, between 1899 and 1913 real wages declined by about 10 per cent and between 1906 and 1908 the trade unionists out of work rose from 4 to 8 per cent.[6] At the time when Miss Loane was writing there was real hardship which was to manifest itself in social unrest in 1910, and this was a reason why Associations found it difficult to get payments from patients. Moreover, in 1914, as in the Boer War, the enlisting sergeant was to find that many recruits were unfit by reason of poor health and substandard nutrition. Cooking lessons and leaflets had not been enough. In 1916 Sir George Newman, the Chief Medical Officer at the Board of Education, reported that 'half a million children in elementary schools were suffering from malnutrition, a condition leading directly to disease'.[7]

QUEEN'S NURSES AND THE PUBLIC

Although the pages of the *Queen's Nurses' Magazine* and other journals are full of accounts of events promoted and patronised by ladies — and sometimes gentlemen — of society to raise money to pay for the nurse's salary and the expenses of the Association, and Queen's nurses were offered rest breaks and holidays in 'delightful country houses', in the delicate social fabric of the time the Queen's nurses themselves were often providers of charity. We read of nurses collecting from their family and friends and organising jumble sales partly to help the poor mothers, and also to raise money for the Association. In poor urban areas the Queen's nurses organised a Christmas party for the poor and especially the crippled children in their district, providing the traditional Father Christmas, oranges and presents out of their own money or from gifts from friends. Queen's nurses were often a special part of the social fabric of the poor. Scotland and Ireland seemed particularly strong on this score, possibly because communities were more closeknit.

One nurse reported starting a library for convalescent patients, partly no doubt to fulfil what Miss Hughes described as the true mission of a Queen's nurse 'to raise them [the patients] to a higher level' but no doubt from goodness of heart to relieve the tedium of the sick. The same enterprising lady reported hiring a 'pony and low chaise to take a detachment of old men and women for a drive when she was free on Saturday afternoon', and she played her violin to 'the old chronics'. Life on the district was bound up with the community and clearly there was not much distinction between 'on duty' and 'off duty'.[8]

The fact that the Queen's nurses had a special regard in the public esteem is summed up in a leading article in *The Times* in 1908. It is an appeal for funds for the Institute, and, after a brief history of Queen Victoria's benefaction, it states that district nursing:

is women's work for women, domestic work, silent, unobtrusive remote from the noise of politics and the turmoil of the market place . . . It is in the homes of the poor, it moves on a footing of peculiar intimacy and sympathy without a trace of condescension. . . . But when one looks at what she [the Queen's nurse] does, and what the suffragettes do, for instance, one seems to be looking at a Bedlam full of shrieking maniacs besides some sane, sober workman going on quietly with useful work.[9]

The leader writer, no doubt a man, liked to portray nurses as womanly women not interfering in a man's world; the comparison served the chauvinistic cause. It is, however, doubtful if this is how the leaders of the Queen's nurses wished to be portrayed; the journals show they were ardently interested in public issues. In 1911 district nurses were asking for an investigation by the Home Secretary into 'the indecent behaviour on the part of the police in their dealings with suffragettes'. One writer, commenting on the complaint by a male writer about women enjoying the prestige of modern advancement and being wedded to their profession instead of becoming mothers, wrote: 'While men think and talk in this strain is it to be wondered that they are hardly acceptable husbands to women whose mental equipment is on another plane of development'.[10] Evidently not all district nurses were womanly women.

QUEEN'S NURSES AND THE MEDICAL PROFESSION

The public and *The Times* may have been loud in their praise of the new 'trained district nurse' but that admiration was not always shared by the medical profession. The antagonism to nurses in the community had been exacerbated by the Midwives Act of 1902, against which the doctors had fought long and hard. In 1908 the Penwith Medical Union in Penzance complained that district nurses were attending minor ailments and treating cuts, thus depriving doctors of their living. They also complained that it was reversing the order of things for a nurse to send for a doctor; the doctor should send for the nurse and she should obey *his* orders. Doctors were trained in hospitals where nursing, in its desire to become academic, had adopted the medical model and on the wards nurses were the doctor's assistants, but in the community nurses were prescribing nursing care. In a letter to the Queen's Institute, Dr Whitaker of the British Medical Association suggested that the two groups should meet and draw up rules. This meeting took place and the BMA set out its proposed rules which included an elaborate system of payment from patients, for if the patient could be made to pay enough for a nurse they would not be so reluctant to call a doctor. The other main rule was to be that the nurse should only attend a case if sanctioned by a doctor. The BMA then went on to propose regulations that were the province of the Institute; for example, nurses were not to wear ornaments, their hours of duty should be prescribed and, an ironical touch, nurses were not to accept presents from patients. There is no evidence that this rule was applied to its own members. History does not relate how the representatives of the Institute dealt with these proposals, but presumably the BMA was referred to the articles of the Charter. Dr Whitaker, apparently not mollified, pointed out:

> the weapon in the hands of the medical profession was a strike, and the refusal to attend cases with nurses and that resolutions to this effect had been adopted by some societies. The central body of the BMA hoped that by conference it might be possible to avoid such a step.[11]

In the end wiser counsels prevailed. The situation was discussed at the Annual Meeting of the BMA in 1909 and one representative pointed out that in places like the Western Isles there was no doctor, and the rules proposed would prevent poor people from having the services of a nurse. Part of the anxiety of the doctors lay in what was later to be called the extended duties of the nurse; under the rules of the Central Midwives Board a midwife was allowed to administer aperients, ergot and anodynes on her own responsibility; where, asked some doctors, would this stop? There was discussion about the nurse being responsible for her own acts, thus implying that the nurse had a professional responsibility. However, delegates in the end took a less belligerent attitude and a strike was not called. Nevertheless, the controversy rankled on, though shortages of nurses and doctors during the First World War healed some wounds, but the dispute reared its head again during the depression of the 1930s when some doctors were having difficulty in making ends meet, and it had not entirely died out by the beginning of the health service.

However warm the public appreciation, and however antagonistic the medical profession, one thing was clear: there was a severe shortage of district nurses in many areas, although in others there was overlapping by various organisations including religious societies and parish nurses. Dr Shadwell, a member of Council speaking at a conference in 1911,[12] said that district nursing, like all voluntary movements, had developed in a haphazard and irregular way. Now the Midwives Act, the Education Act and the National Insurance Act meant that there was an increased demand for district nurses, and Associations were brought into contact with public authorities. Unfortunately, the Queen's Institute had not the power to speak for its own Associations, or other bodies, nor to conduct negotiations on their behalf. What the Queen's Institute needed was popular democratic backing to carry weight in a modern world. This, however, was the difficulty: the Institute had only a tenuous hold over its affiliates, who were often run by the most powerful members of society and it had no hold over other district nursing associations. All too soon, however, the spate of conferences on the future of health care provision were forgotten as attention was diverted to the Irish question and the growing menace of a European war.

NURSES DURING THE FIRST WORLD WAR

In 1914 there were 2100 nurses on the Queen's Roll and some of these were on the reserve of the Queen Alexandra Imperial Military Nursing Service or other organisations, and many others volunteered. In the first year of the war 652 Queen's Nurses were called up leaving the service desperately short of trained nurses. Replacement for training was not forthcoming from hospitals because of the rush to volunteer to nurse the wounded. In vain, superintendents went round the hospitals lecturing on the importance of district nursing. One voiced a *cri du coeur* to be echoed by many a latter-day nursing officer for the community.

> Some matrons are interested, a few are out of sympathy altogether. Most are ignorant of what district nurses do and of their training and they think they are lost forever. The nurses themselves are not responsive, they are too tired.[13]

On the credit side the *Queen's Nurses' Magazine* was able to report that thanks to wartime employment there was now less poverty. Superintendents reported that 'in nutrition, cleanliness, and in health the condition of the children compared favourably with those examined in past years and in clothing and foot gear they were better'. At the same time there had been a diminution of crime 'proving once more, were proof required, that the removal of the great curse of unemployment is the remedy to be applied in the future for the permanent improvement of social conditions'.[14]

While those left behind battled on with the new duties imposed upon them for child life protection and maternity and child welfare regulations their colleagues were sending home accounts of their exploits abroad. Many Queen's nurses were called up on short-term contracts, but it says much for the comprehensiveness of the training and for the sheer hardiness and resilience of the Queen's nurses themselves that so many played such an important part in military service. Used to cycling miles across the bogs of Ireland, taking boats to the Outer Hebrides, improvising in cottages and putting cellars in nursing order, they seemed to take to active service like ducks to water. From the accounts in the journals, a number seem to have gone out with the Serbian Relief Fund. One group described their journey from the Mersey menaced all the time by submarines, an experience to be repeated by nurses of the next generation. Working by candlelight and dealing with typhus was not a new experience, but coping with the Serbian language was. When the typhus patients began to fall off and life became calmer, with the help of French doctors, the nurses started a baby clinic and dispensary for the destitute and stricken Serbian mothers. Miss Coaling, the superintendent of Queen's nurses from Southampton, wrote a pamphlet 'Hints to Mothers' which was translated into various languages and printed in Serbian and, with her nurses, ran a maternity and child welfare clinic. The enterprise was not without danger because the hospital was bombarded, but in spite of this the party say 'they left Serbia with many regrets'.[15]

Miss Tylecote, another Queen's nurse, was one of the last to tramp over the mountains on the retreat back to Salonika, during which time she developed scarlet fever. She journeyed on plunging through icy rivers, sleeping in wet clothes, and in a graphic article she describes how the party bivouacked in any village that would have them, and the sheer joy of finding a fire where they could dry their clothes and fry their tinned bacon then, 'sleeping on the mud floor the party were refreshed and ready to climb the mountain paths again'. The journey took several weeks during which time they were lost, often short of food, the going was hard and often hazardous, but presumably they reached Salonika because the article says laconically 'Miss Tylecote arrived safely in England just before Christmas'.[15]

Yet another group of nurses including Queen's nurses, were taken prisoner by the Austrians. Fortunately, their captors were 'polite and treated them well'. Their experiences as prisoners of war do not seem to have been too harsh and although they spent Christmas under guard they managed to improvise Christmas decorations and festivities, both religious and secular, to the delight of their mixed fellow prisoners and captors. Eventually they were released and returned to England via Switzerland, sleeping in trucks in railway sidings.[16]

Other reports came from Queen's nurses working with units in France, Belgium and India, but an account from Russia is particularly interesting as a reminder of British involvement in, and aid to, that country before the revolution. A Queen's nurse sent a graphic description of her life working on the Steppes of Russia.

I have travelled the Steppes in all weathers and seen them in all conditions; I have heard the wolves and been in snowstorms. A call comes and you go off, the doctor needs your help, it may take a few hours or many to travel there and you may have to stay all night.[17]

In spite of the hardships Miss Graveson loved her work and was expecting to go by sledge in a day or two to start a hospital in Mergslova and put it in nursing order.

Apart from the fact that these women were obviously intrepid, enterprising and hardy, one is impressed by the fact that many of them managed to communicate in a variety of languages and some were good linguists. Moreover, district nurses they may have been, and hospital matrons wondered what they did, but they were capable of setting up and organising hospitals and displaying a capacity for leadership among their colleagues. What is more they wrote well and vividly.

Many Queen's nurses were decorated for their services, and others sent home accounts of torpedo attacks and ordeal by life-boat, some, alas, died, but meanwhile at home all was far from quiet. There is an account of the Silvertown bombing which is reminiscent of the Second World War, and in Shoreditch the Queen's nurses volunteered to the Red Cross Hospital Ambulance Column which met every train of wounded arriving in London. This meant that the nurses often gave up a night's rest because calls mostly came at night, and before returning to their day duties they spent their time dealing with the most harrowing sights.

Life on the district went on. The realities of war, the influx of the Voluntary Aid Detachment (VAD), the use of auxiliaries and village nurses to fill the gaps again raised the question that had been smouldering for years: should trained nurses be registered? The Queen's nurses debated the question. In earlier rounds of that frenzied argument, the Queen's Institute, secure in its own badge and certificate, was inclined to take the Nightingale view that nursing was 'about living spirits' and that registration would be meaningless. Now, however, Miss Nightingale was dead and the war had changed the situation; it seemed the public as well as the profession needed protection.

In the midst of the controversy, in 1916, the Hon. Arthur Stanley, secretary to the Joint War Organisation, together with Dame Sarah Swift, lately matron of Guy's Hospital, launched an appeal for the foundation of a College of Nursing: 'to unite all nurses in overcoming the many differences of opinion among nurses themselves . . .

with the task of coordinating the whole profession'. Queen's nurses were urged to join the new organisation and make sure it was representative of the profession. 'On Queen's nurses especially do we think there is laid an obligation. Ever since they joined the Queen's Institute they have known — in a lesser degree — the advantages that State Registration offers to all nurses'.[18] At this juncture, of course, it was envisaged that the new College would be the registering body.

The appeal did not fall on deaf ears. The activities of the College were soon being advertised in the pages of the *Queen's Nurses' Magazine* and many Queen's nurses became members, often playing an important part in the work of the public health section when it was formed. As workers in the wider world, the Queen's nurses often saw the need for the development of nursing as a profession more clearly than did their sisters in hospital.

HEALTH VISITORS AND MIDWIVES

One aspect of the development of nursing that concerned the Queen's Institute deeply was that of the emergence of the health visitor, whose activities had been validated by the Notification of Births Act and who had a recognised training and an examination by the Royal Sanitary Institute. From the articles in the nursing press it is clear that there was considerable friction between the midwives and the new health visitors, and, of course, the district nurses saw themselves as the true health missionaries. No one seems to have thought it worthwhile to hammer out a demarcation of duties, and, indeed, who was to do it? There was no Ministry of Health, no nursing council and the College of Nursing was too new. Undoubtedly, some Medical Officers of Health issued ill-advised regulations and health visitors were overlapping with, and clashing with, midwives, some of whom, in spite of their new status, were not versed in the art of child welfare.

Resentment was felt because health visitors sometimes visited the patient while the midwife was in attendance on the pretext of seeing if there was a risk of ophthalmia neonatorum, and worse still, the inspection of midwives was sometimes given to 'young and inexperienced health visitors'. It has to be remembered that some health visitors were university graduates and some were women doctors. Reading between the lines there was resentment that the health visitors were 'well paid by the ratepayer and had little responsibility and shorter hours of work' than the 'ill-paid midwife up all hours of the day and night'. The older midwives and district nurses resented the new young women with their certificates, college training and new ideas; the better educated resented them because they wanted to extend their empire to all fields of public health.

Meanwhile there was friction between the Queen's nurses and midwives, and conferences discussed whether or not Queen's nurses should in fact be involved in midwifery. Was midwifery an entirely separate profession? But as one writer put it:

At the moment midwives and health visitors seem inclined to wear the hedgehog's coat and to be full of prickles, but as both exist for the welfare of mothers and babies we must hope that ere long misunderstanding will disappear and harmony will prevail. Of all workers these two should be allies not enemies.[19]

The hope was a pious one. The lack of any standard as to who was a trained nurse, the confusion as to whether the midwife should first be a nurse, the unfortunate historical image of the midwife, the doubtful area of the health visitor's responsibility, the difference in the organisations, and their status, employing district nurses, the various lines of accountability of the different workers and the difference in the reward all led to confusion and suspicion made worse by the divorce between curative and preventive medicine. The attitude in nursing only mirrored the attitudes of medicine, where traditional hospital doctors and general practitioners regarded medical officers in public health with suspicion.

The confusion and distrust cast long shadows before them to darken many attempts to unify and reform both the basic and post basic nurse training. Those who are concerned with the fissiparous nature of nursing and the hedgehog coats that were so manifest after the report of the Committee on Nursing in 1970, should look at the pages of the nursing journals for the First World War.

NOTES

1. The Poor Law Commission, Minority Report, HMSO, 1909.

2. Report and Proceedings of the Jubilee Congress of District Nursing 1909, Liverpool, D. Marples, p. 199.

3. Conference on the National Insurance Act, Denison House, Westminster, 28 February 1912.

4. *The Daily Chronicle* on the second impression of *Neighbours and Friends* quoted in Edward Arnold's Spring Announcement 1909.

5. Loane, M. *The Queen's Poor*, Edward Arnold, London, third

impression 1909, p. 136.

6. Cole, G.D. and Postgate, R. *The Common People*, 4th edn, Methuen, London, 1949, p. 498.

7. The Report of the Chief Medical Officer of Health, Board of Education 1915–1916, HMSO, London.

8. *Queen's Nurses' Magazine*, 1 May 1904, p. 16.

9. *The Times*, leading article, 23 March 1908.

10. *Nursing Notes*, 11 September 1911.

11. Minutes of a meeting held between representatives of the BMA and the Queen's Institute, 8 March 1909.

12. Proceedings of Conference on the Effect of the National Insurance Act on Interested Organisations, 24 May 1911.

13. *Queen's Nurses' Magazine*, Impressions of a Traveller, January 1914.

14. *Queen's Nurses' Magazine*, editorial, January 1916, pp. 1–2.

15. *Queen's Nurses' Magazine*, With the Hospitals in Serbia, January 1916, pp. 6 and 9.

16. *Queen's Nurses' Magazine*, A Prisoner in Serbia, January 1917, p. 3.

17. *Queen's Nurses' Magazine*, News from Russia, April 1917, p. 33.

18. *Queen's Nurses' Magazine*, editorial, July 1916, p. 60.

19. *Queen's Nurses' Magazine*, A Note on Health Visiting, July 1916, p. 69.

7

The World We Have Lost

At the beginning of the First World War the Queen's Jubilee Institute had 2096 nurses on the Roll. In 1919 there were only 1999, and more tasks had been added to the work of the district nurse. In spite of the 2577 health visitors now employed, district nurses had become more involved with maternity and child welfare, with tuberculosis nursing, and there was much overlapping of duties. The *Queen's Nurses' Magazine* in an editorial pinpointed the problem that was to grow with the years and which did not disappear with the National Health Service or any of its reorganisations: 'The problem of the multiplicity of remedial agencies now in being for the benefit of the sick poor, with all and each of which the district nurse comes in touch in the course of her daily round'.[1]

To add to the problems of the shortage of nurses and war weariness came the devastating influenza epidemic in the autumn of 1918, the descriptions of which, coming in from the districts, sometimes sound like those of the great plague: 'we had to superintend the removal of the dead before we could start nursing the living'.

With no effective treatment available the epidemic took a high toll of young adults: 'in some cases the eyes swelled and burst and the patient died in acute suffering. In other cases there would be an acute form of stomatitis, the tongue, the uvulae and the soft parts sloughing away in spite of constant treatment'.[2]

The district nurses toiled away as best they could and sadly a number died as the result of the infection, losses the Institute could ill afford. In 1919 ten district nurses died, 324 resigned and only 121 new nurses were placed on the Roll.

LEGACIES OF THE FIRST WORLD WAR

The reasons for the shortage of district nurses were discussed at length in the journals and at conferences, some of which were to appear on district nursing conferences' agenda for the next 50 or so years. These included the reluctance of trained nurses to face another training and to bind themselves to a contract, the fear of loneliness after the rush of hospital life, the general ignorance of district nursing and what it entailed and, above all, the inadequate salary, lack of pensions and no real leisure time.[3]

Contrary to expectations, fewer women were now taking up nursing: the wave of altruism was over. At the same time hospitals needed more nurses because more people were using hospitals and the hours nurses worked there, though still long, were shorter. There was a tendency for women who wished to work to look for other opportunities, and because of trade union pressure in industry women who had worked now returned to domestic life. The battle for liberation from the kitchen sink had to be won all over again in the Second World War.

Because of the war and the fall in donations, the Institute was in desperate straits for money. In order to attract recruits they needed to offer a salary of £63 to £75 a year with £10 for uniform and 25 shillings a week for board and lodging, but many associations could not afford this. In 1920 the College of Nursing published recommended salaries for all grades of nurses which suggested a salary of £85 to £120 a year for resident district nurses. This was not princely; in 1920 a bricklayer, if in work, could earn £5 a week. The paradox for the Institute was that district nurses were most needed in the poorest districts. Although, as the Institute noted, there was less primary poverty than in 1914 because wages had risen, prices had also risen and 'there were pockets of hardship, real and imagined, which combined to make 1919 a year of strikes'.[4] This made Provident schemes difficult to administer; a levy on wages was suggested — dangerously near state intervention — but what of the unemployed and the strike-bound? The question of paid collectors was frequently debated, but many questioned whether this was money well spent. Flag days and house-to-house collections abounded and local authorities were asked for more money. But here was the rub: in that embrace what demands for control might come?

War is a test of institutions, provoking their dissolution or transformation, and because of shared sacrifice by different groups there is an increase in the expectation for greater equality of treatment.

The First World War was total war and it tested institutions in a way no other war had done. War was the sorcerer's apprentice, the genie let out of the bottle never to be returned.

One result of the shared sacrifice by women was the extension of the franchise to include women over the age of 30 years — on the reckoning that by the age of 30 women had the maturity of men of 21 years. This is not to devalue the efforts of the suffragettes, but after the war only the most chauvinistic males could hold out. Regardless of the 'womanly work' image beloved in propaganda when collecting funds for Queen's nurses, the *Queen's Nurses' Magazine* was quick to urge its readers to use their votes if they had one and watch new developments about the provision of health care with an eagle eye.

Another consequence of the war was the promise of a better and more equitable health service. A committee under Sir Donald Maclean with Beatrice Webb on one of the subcommittees recommended the breakup of the Poor Law and the transfer of all health matters, including nursing, to the counties and county boroughs. In 1919 Lloyd George was returned at the head of a coalition government with a manifesto that included the implementation of the Maclean report. Well may the *Queen's Nurses' Magazine* have warned its readers to watch events. As it happened, the protest from the medical profession and the Local Government Board was so strong that the Bill was withdrawn. However, some progress was made, the Local Government Board was swept away and a Ministry of Health was set up with Dr Addison, a Liberal MP as the first Minister of Health. A Council on Medical and Administrative Services was set up under Dr Bernard Dawson (later Lord Dawson of Penn) which recommended the creation of health authorities to combine curative and preventive practice from which would work doctors, nurses, midwives and health visitors. The scheme was widely discussed but it ran into opposition: first, from medical officers of health who felt that the general practitioners had no training in preventive medicine, an opinion with which the health visitors probably agreed; second, from the doctors themselves who saw it as a precursor to state medicine; and finally, from the voluntary organisations who feared for their donations. In any event, as the postwar depression hit the country and unemployment rose, there was no hope of financing the scheme, and it and Dr Addison were quietly dropped. The doctors and nurses settled down to flag days and the *status quo ante*, and the Ministry of Health to very little control over the health services of the country. An indication of the economic slump can be seen in a letter from the Institute to its district nursing associations. Contrary to what was to happen in the 1980s, high unemployment led to a fall in prices and to deflation; because of this in 1922 the Institute was able to suggest that associations paid their nurses a *lower* allowance for board and lodging, an invitation which they no doubt needed no second bidding to accept.[5]

A further outcome of the war was the state registration of nurses. The College of Nursing with representatives of the Queen's Institute pressed for registration, as did other organisations such as the Royal British Nurses' Association led by Mrs Bedford Fenwick. The war had changed the situation, now it was the public which needed to be protected from the hosts of 'amateur' nurses who had swelled the war-time ranks. In the unseemly row that followed, with different organisations pressing for different standards, the Minister of Health intervened and set up his own statutory body, the General Nursing Council.[6] Thanks to its internecine warfare, the nursing profession handed the control of its basic training to the government who, of course, had a vested interest in keeping down costs. The new Council did not innovate but fixed nurse training with legislation in the groove it had developed so far; it did nothing to widen the basic training, and the gap between the hospital and the community was as wide as ever. However, Miss Peterkin, the Queen's Institute Superintendent, was on the Council and soon Queen's nurses were being urged to register and eventually state registration became the *sine qua non* for acceptance for Queen's training.

DISTRICT NURSES AND HEALTH VISITORS

Meanwhile, the confusion of the roles of district nurses and health visitors continued. Examinations for the Queen's Roll continued to ask questions that related to health teaching and the running of welfare centres. Medical officers, when asked by questionnaire, expressed a variety of views as to who should perform such tasks, some preferring Queen's nurses, others saying that a special training was necessary.[7] However, the new Ministry of Health took the matter in hand and issued a circular outlining the duties of a health visitor which included maternity and child welfare work and the school medical services, and went on to suggest that persons undertaking this work should undergo a special training.

It is fully recognised that the three years' training for a fully qualified nurse or the training for the certificate of the CMB is of value to the health visitor, but these do not cover the many functions the health visitor is expected to perform.[8]

In 1919 the Ministry of Health together with the Board of Education promulgated a scheme for training health visitors. There were to be three methods of entry: by post-basic training for a person who was a qualified nurse; by a year's training for a person who was a university graduate; and by two years' training for a person who was neither a nurse nor a graduate. It has been argued that if this imaginative approach had been followed much of the subsequent controversy about social works, their types and which sex they were would have been avoided.[9] However, the great concern of the new Ministry of Health was the infant mortality rate, for although this had fallen to 51 per 1000 live births, it was recognised that there were many avoidable deaths; in 1925 a new circular laid down that in future all entrants to health visitor training must have six months' training in midwifery. This, of course, determined that health visitors should be women; it also limited the number of Queen's nurses eligible to take the course. It was also decided that the Royal Sanitary Institute, founded in 1876, should be the examining body for the Certificate of Health Visiting, and that the Ministry of Health should be responsible for approving training centres. The Queen's Institute hoped that it would be approved for training, but the Ministry deemed that the course needed to be more academic and to have a different emphasis. Therefore, 1925 marks a divide between district nursing and health visiting, a divide that was to have consequences for the development and the relationship of the two services. Some Queen's nurses who were suitable, seeing the attraction of the higher salary paid by the local authorities, took the training and became health visitors, others took the training and returned to work under the auspices of the Institute to perform triple duties in rural areas for which they were paid from a variety of complicated sources.

But training cost money and the Institute prepared to launch another national appeal. Unfortunately this coincided with the great postwar fund-raising appeal for all nurses by Lady Cowdray, on behalf of the Nation's Fund for Nurses, which, after much diplomacy and counter-diplomacy, included the Queen's Institute as one of its beneficiaries. In spite of high hopes and victory balls the fund did not raise the money expected, and for the time the Queen's Institute was obliged to abandon some part of its training and inspection. The wolf was snarling at the door. If the Institute could not afford nurses who would bring it credit and prestige it would surely disappear.

Help came, as it had done in 1901, by a royal death. Queen Alexandra, a much loved patron of nurses, died and in 1926 a meeting was called at the Mansion House to inaugurate a Memorial Fund for the Queen's Institute, of which she had long been the patron. Once again committees were organised, appeals were made on the new BBC and by 1928 £233 114 had been raised. The same year saw a new charter for the Institute, and its transformation into the Queen's Institute of District Nursing. The charter defined its objects as being: 'The training, maintenance and supply of women to act as nurses and midwives for the sick poor and for the undertaking of preventive and supervisory work for the securing of their health and the health of their children'.[10] In 1933 the Queen's Institute moved to its present premises in 57 Lower Belgrave Street.

SUPERANNUATION SCHEMES

In 1925 a new scheme was organised and affiliated associations were asked to contribute to a Long Service Fund. Under this arrangement associations paid three pounds for each nurse a year, and after 21 years' service with the Institute, nurses, subject to a means test, were able to receive a small pension. This scheme remained in existence until 1944. In 1928, after negotiations by the College of Nursing, the Federated Superannuation Scheme for Nurses was established, by which the employee paid in a percentage of his or her earnings and the employer paid a percentage contribution with benefits paid on an actuarial basis. Many voluntary hospitals participated and local authority hospitals often had their own schemes. Unfortunately, district nursing associations did not feel able to participate and this produced a further gap between the incentive to hospital work and district nursing. Throughout the early 1930s a recurring theme of the Public Health Section of the College of Nursing was a resolution requesting that the Ministry of Health ensure that the Federated Superannuation Scheme be adopted for all public health nurses.[11]

However, all was not hardship. The *Queen's Nurses' Magazine* frequently advertised holidays: nurses sent back accounts of enterprising holidays abroad; patrons occasionally put part of their country homes at the disposal of Queen's nurses wishing 'to avail themselves of a fortnight's rest free of charge under the most pleasant conditions . . . (references required)';[12] and the Queen's nurses, always internationally minded, attended the Congresses of the International Council of Nurses and sent home reports. In 1911 a Miss

Harriet Hughes bequeathed Bryn-y-Menai, a beautiful house above the Menai Strait, to the Institute as a home of rest for Queen's nurses and many a district nurse found solace there until it was closed in 1947.

THE INTERWAR YEARS

The central issue of the interwar years was undoubtedly unemployment. Often this was associated with sickness, and while on the one hand this made demands on the district nursing service, on the other it decreased the possibility of collecting subscriptions. In 1929 Neville Chamberlain, now Minister of Health, introduced his Local Government Act which swept away the old Boards of Guardians, and local authorities were urged to set up Public Assistance Committees for the relief of destitution. The new committees were responsible for the old Poor Law functions of welfare, health, the disabled and pauper children. However, in spite of high hopes that some of the principles of the Maclean report would be implemented, most people saw the new Public Assistance Committees as the old Poor Law writ large, and the Institute was no more successful in wresting money from them for district nursing than it had been from the Boards of Guardians. Among the poor, tuberculosis nursing became a heavy commitment for district nurses, and in 1931 there were 992 deaths per million population from that preventible disease.

After the Local Government Act the London County Council asked Dr Margaret Hogarth to carry out a survey of district nursing in London and to see what steps it needed to take. Her report stresses the value of the work being done by voluntary organisations; of the 32 district nursing associations, 22 working from 24 nurses' homes, were affiliated to the Queen's Institute.

> From what I have seen of the work of these nurses in the homes, I do not consider that the educational and preventive effect of a nursing visit can be over-estimated. In this connection I am of the opinion that for any domiciliary nursing of patients under the new arrangements the services of these nursing organisations should be retained and that a district nurse should be present at each medical session at district offices or dispensaries.[13]

The London County Council retained the use of the voluntary organisations on an agency basis and many other local authorities did the same.

Unemployment

The depression of the early 1930s, the high unemployment and the difficulties of many doctors earning a living in areas of high deprivation rekindled some of the old animosity between doctors and nurses. Although most Queen's nurses were scrupulous in obeying the doctor's orders, and often had a happy relationship with doctors, it was not always so. In 1932 there was correspondence in the *British Medical Journal* referring to the sheltered life of the Medical Officer of Health, the *bête noir* of some general practitioners. An enraged 'GP' wrote

> He and the general public who enjoy promoting philanthropic institutions [district nurses] ought to realise that the general practitioner has a hard job to pay rates, taxes and school fees, if he can afford children. The district nurse now takes most of his midwifery, does ante-natal and post-natal work and during these visits is consulted on every ailment which she diagnoses and treats. If she does not she is told they will not contribute their pence to the Association. . . . She does minor surgery, sends patients to hospital for advice and treatment. She takes stitches out of the perineum without sanction and if asked to massage a fracture is 'untrained' or too busy with her confinement cases. . . . In other words she is one of the GP's most dangerous opponents.[14]

The correspondence continued, some letters agreeing but with others rushing to declare a happy relationship with the nurses 'under his control' (*sic*). No doubt a few district nurses were tactless, but what the correspondence highlights is not so much demarcation disputes, but the tensions of the times with doctors scraping for a living and nurses scraping for contributions, a situation that by 1938 made even the *British Medical Association* contemplate the possibility, and the benefits of, a national health service.

In 1932 22.1 per cent of the working population were unemployed. Nine ministers resigned over cuts in unemployment benefit, income tax rose to 5 shillings in the pound, public services were asked to take cuts of 10 per cent in their pay, and the gold standard was suspended. All this concentrated the mind wonderfully. If you had a job the great thing was to remain in it. In spite of this, it was alleged that nursing was failing to attract recruits in the numbers and of the quality needed. In 1930 the proprietors of *The Lancet* set up a

Commission to enquire into the shortages of candidates for nursing the sick and to offer suggestions. It happened that the College of Nursing was contemplating its own inquiry and the two bodies cooperated closely.[15] Miss Wilmshurst, the General Superintendent of the Queen's Institute, was on the delegation from the College. The Commission came to the conclusion, though on scant evidence, that nursing was falling into disfavour as an occupation, and it made suggestions for improving it, and these included implementing the scales of money laid down by the College and improving living conditions for nurses. On the subject of district nursing the Commission had this to say:

> The pay of the district nurse is outside our terms of reference except in so far as it is one of the prospects ultimately open to probationers. The efforts of the Nursing Associations to obtain funds are so valiant and the needs of the services so manifest that it is with reluctance that we state our conviction that the pay offered in this field is inadequate. The district nurse is the general practitioner of nursing and so deserves a salary that will enable her to command some comfort in her home . . . .[16]

The *Lancet* report was widely discussed in the nursing journals including the *Queen's Nurses' Magazine*, but as the voluntary hospitals struggled for donations, sometimes literally to repair the roof over their heads, and the affiliated nursing associations rattled their collecting boxes there was little hope of improving the financial lot of nurses, though there was some examination of outmoded discipline.

Midwifery

In spite of the exhortation for Queen's nurses to use their midwifery training, midwifery was not undertaken to any large extent by nursing associations in towns. For the most part midwives worked as independent practitioners under the local supervising authority; but in spite of improvements, the maternal mortality rate of 2.56 per 1000 births was unacceptably high, and in 1936 a Bill was introduced to bring midwives under the aegis of the local authority as a salaried service. The Queen's Institute welcomed the Bill because: 'it [the Bill] recognised there was already a satisfactory service in connection with training hospitals and Nursing Associations under the Queen's Institute. It was not intended to interfere with voluntary bodies but to help independent midwives.[17] The Institute in fact saw the Bill as a way to extend their midwifery services and it was, of course, another way of collecting payments from local authorities.

Ireland and Scotland

In 1921 a treaty had given dominion status to Ireland apart from the six counties that were given limited self-government, and the Irish Free State was proclaimed in 1922. In spite of this, the Institute continued to have branches in Ireland and received reports of ingenious money-raising activities and hair-raising accounts of boat trips to emergencies in storms off the Aran Isles. All, however, was not work. There were weekend visits:

> We came back to Mrs Somerville, Bantry, Joint Hon Secretary at 3.30 pm and played tennis, putting etc until 6.30 pm, had a very nice tea. That evening there was a dance in one of the hotels and we went for a few hours. We enjoyed it very much.[18]

The news from Scotland was less about tea and dances and more about the rigours of nursing in the highlands and islands, and the problems of improvising in the But and Ben and of ever reaching one's destination. Reports from Scotland show how the maternity and child welfare movement had taken root there, and described the progress of training centres and the cooperation with health visitors. But over all the reports from Scotland and Ireland comes the message of terrible poverty and interwar unemployment; depression that was to cause a wave of emigration and problems for the post-Second World War world. A recurring theme from Scotland is of the parties given by nurses themselves for their poorer patients, especially for the poor and crippled children. Charity as a word had not lost its Pauline beauty.

Not only were there Queen's nurses being rowed to the Outer Hebrides and being storm-tossed off the coast of Ireland, there were Queen's nurses on the Channel Isles. Two had started a service there in 1910 and by the outbreak of the Second World War there were sixteen. The stories of those who stayed throughout the occupation often on starvation rations compare with their sisters of an earlier generation who braved the rivers of Serbia.

There were advantages

In spite of low pay, lack of pensions, long hours and the often con-
descending attitude of hospitals to district work the Queen's Institute
did attract recruits for the simple reason that many found it a satisfying life, more satisfying than the discipline and the cloistered existence
of institutional life. On the district the nurse was part of the community, she was a citizen with a life of her own. For all the hardship
of the interwar years many district nurses remembered it as a world
we have lost.

For a while, before the introduction of antibiotics, much illness
depended on skilled nursing. Medicine could often do little for the
pneumonia or typhoid patient, but skilled nursing could do much and
this was recognised by the public, and often acknowledged by the
doctors. The district nurses saved lives. But more than that, before
the age of so much specialisation, in a rural area the well-trained
district nurse could encompass many roles and be the guide,
philosopher and friend of the neighbourhood. If she was triply trained,
as a midwife she often saw women through pregnancy and delivery,
as a health visitor she advised on infant feeding and the care of the
toddler whom she knew when he went to the village school. She gave
talks to adolescents and visited the grandparents. She was everybody's
friend. Medicine was such that one person, suitably trained, could
possess all the skills required.

On the physical side the world we have lost had its consolations.
The salary may have been low but the District Association often
stipulated that the nurse should have 'attendance'. Inspectors com-
mented if the nurse had no daily help or landlady to care for her,
and the pages of the *Queen's Nurses' Magazine* are full of delightful
stories about the trials — or blessings — of landladies and daily maids
who were kept waiting while the nurse was called out.

Transport and the district nurse

Although many a nurse still did her rounds on her bicycle, motor cars
and motor cycles were coming into vogue, and if a rural association
really wanted a nurse it had to offer a car. In 1928 Dorset had six
cars and nine motor cycles, by 1933 there were 24 motor cars, ten
of which were owned by nurses themselves — this at a time when
car ownership really was a status symbol. In 1932 Cornwall only had
eight cars, but by the outbreak of the war this had risen to 62.

However, there was a marked divide between north and south; in 1933 Sunderland had only one car.[19] The motor car transformed district nursing; it meant that greater distances could be covered, emergencies dealt with more quickly, more equipment carried and the nurse arrived dry. The car was money well spent. There were no traffic wardens, no yellow lines, no parking problems, and except for the vagaries of double declutching and the hazards of the early models, the nurse who drove a car was wonderfully free. Before mass transport, high technology farming and commuting transformed rural life the Queen's nurse enjoyed a special prestige. Maybe the funds for the district association to pay her salary had to be met by the village fête or jumble sales, but this was all part of the pattern of life; after all, the local hospital was kept going by the same voluntary effort. It was, of course, an unequal society, but that was relative to what had gone before, and in that unequal society the Queen's nurses had a place.

Whether this was a satisfactory life obviously depended on the temperament and the professional ability of the nurse herself. In spite of the condescension of posterity, many Queen's nurses recall these years with pleasure and many seem to have found a niche in that subtle hierarchy of rural life that was the hallmark of the interwar years and that now can only be glimpsed through the films of the period or television series.

In the towns the provision of the much-coveted car was rare; moreover, there was more specialisation: health visitors ran welfare clinics and visited the toddlers, there was probably a separately employed school nurse, the midwife was employed by the local authority as were the social workers. To some extent the district nurse was out on a limb, and the different nursing groups may have had little contact with one another unless they met at branch meetings of the College of Nursing. With the increasing use of hospitals in the 1930s — and this was the heyday of the 'cottage hospital' — fewer tonsils were removed on the kitchen table and doctors were more inclined to refer patients to hospital. District nursing gradually changed; and there was greater emphasis on long-term care and those illnesses consultants wrote off as 'not suitable for this hospital', which meant incurable and therefore uninteresting, and which, of course, were all too often the cases requiring the most nursing. To some extent it slowly became a self-fulfilling prophecy; the district nurse was sent the 'chronic' cases, and in time hospitals thought these were all she was capable of nursing.

The bicycle, the motor car and above all the motor cycle forced a change of uniform on the nurses of the Institute, though not without some misgivings, for the bonnet and cloak had become a symbol similar to the bearskins of the Guards. Gradually the pages of the journals are full of advertisements for smart frock coats that become shorter as the years go by, the storm cap was introduced in the same material as the coat with braid and badge, price 7/9–10/9 (about 50p). A smart gaberdine overcoat (showerproof) cost between £3 and £4 and, in 1936, 'Dora caps in fine lawn for shingled hair' cost 1 shilling and 4½ pence (approximately 7p). However, in spite of exhortations to sartorial excellence, Queen's inspectors continued to write on reports 'uniform not quite correct'.

In towns it was more difficult to be 'not quite correct' because district nurses usually worked from a district nurses' home under the eye of a superintendent, and although after the war there was a rebellion against these, not all were forbidding and cheerless. As the journals show, some district associations took a pride in supplying comforts like central heating and tennis courts that were hard to come by outside, and some provided a comradeship and shared experience that in some ways compensated for the lack of 'a life of your own'. With three million surplus women, unequal pay and limited opportunities for women, the Nurses' Home was, *faute de mieux*, sometimes a cheerful refuge. It was not until the 1960s that a single woman on a modest income could get a mortgage. Above all, district nursing gave nurses the satisfaction of being an independent practitioner free from the shackles of hospital life. As Florence Nightingale said: 'District Nursing, so solitary, so without cheer and stimulus of a big corps of fellow workers in the bustle of a public hospital but [is] also without many of its cares and strains . . .'[20]

NOTES

1. *Queen's Nurses' Magazine*, editorial, August 1919.

2. *Queen's Nurses' Magazine*, February 1919, p. 31.

3. Report of a Conference of Affiliated Associations, England and Wales, 20 July 1920, Lowe Bros, London.

4. Marwick, A. *The Deluge*, Macmillan, London, 1965, p. 272.

5. Queen Victoria's Jubilee Institute/to all Affiliated District Nursing Associations, March 1922.

6. Abel-Smith, B. *A History of the Nursing Profession*, Heinemann, London, 1960, p. 61. See also Baly, M.E. *Nursing and Social Change*, Heinemann, London, 1982, Chapter 12.

7. Reports from County Nursing Officers on reactions of Medical Officers

of Health, April 1917.

8. Ministry of Health circular 1919, quoted in Lamb, A. *Primary Health Nursing*, Ballière and Tindall, London, p. 117.

9. Clarke, J. *A Family Visitor*, RCN, London, 1973, p. 17.

10. The Queen's Institute of District Nursing, Supplemental Charter, 1928.

11. Minutes of the Council of the College of Nursing, January 1931.

12. *Queen's Nurses' Magazine*, Lady FitzGerald's invitation, March 1936, p. 268.

13. *District Nursing in London* (pamphlet). Report of survey carried out by Dr Margaret Hogarth presented to the London County Council, 1929.

14. *British Medical Journal*, 26 March 1932, p. 598.

15. Minutes of the Council of the College of Nursing, February 1931.

16. *Report of the Lancet Commission*, published by the *Lancet*, 1932.

17. *Queen's Nurses' Magazine*, September 1936, editorial, pp. 329 and 355.

18. *Queen's Nurses' Magazine*, 1936, p. 355.

19. Public Records' Office, Inspectors' Reports, PRO 30/63/93, 54 and 34, 1932, 1933.

20. Miss Nightingale's address to the Metropolitan and National Nursing Association, GLRO HR/ST/NC 15, 13c, 1878.

8

The Coming of the National Health Service

In the First World War Queen's nurses were encouraged to volunteer for the armed services. In 1939 it was feared that the needs of civilians would be greater, and Miss Mercy Wilmshurst, the General Superintendent, sent a message to all Queen's nurses urging them to stay at their posts:

> this may seem less spectacular than that of nursing the wounded whether in the armed services or in the civilian populations . . . but it will win the gratitude of thousands of adults and children who are feeling the separation from home ties keenly.[1]

THE SECOND WORLD WAR

Apart from the exhortation to stay at their posts, in 1943 there was the Control of Engagement Order which meant that nurses could not leave their posts except to take further training. This, however, did not bring the flood of recruits that might have been expected; at the beginning of the war there were 4566 Queen's nurses and at the end 4476; losses more than offset recruitment. Under the chairmanship of Lord Athlone the Queen's Institute continued training nurses and sending out its six inspectors who often worked under great difficulty. Wartime conditions and inflation meant that local associations were unable to raise the same money and there was a decrease in the income from the Gardens Scheme. In 1944 the Council reported that: 'Unless some substantial help is forthcoming it will be impossible to give training to the increasing number of candidates who apply, or carry on the work of the Institute'.[2]

Not for the first, or last, time a subcommittee was set up to effect economies. Fortunately, thanks largely to the untiring efforts of the wartime Council, sufficient money was raised from appeals and charitable events for the work to continue. In 1946, the Chairman of the Gardens Scheme, Hilda, Duchess of Richmond and Gordon, who was an active Council member of the Institute, managed to raise £10 656 and because of such efforts and an increase in the affiliation fees the deficit was reduced. Nevertheless, the Institute entered the era of the National Health Service with a worrying financial position.

During the war district nurses were confronted with new tasks. They met trains and buses, took evacuees to their new homes and looked after schoolchildren. The plight and state of some as described in *Our Towns*[3] showed that all was far from well with the public health of England and was one of the pointers to the need for a more equitable health service after the war. Maternity hospitals and departments were evacuated to the sectors, and district midwives were often hard-pressed with the number of cases undertaken showing a steep rise until 1944 when they fell.[4] As the tide of war ebbed and flowed, so district nurses themselves were evacuated or returned to cities to meet new needs and inspectors' reports cited superintendents as being 'exhausted' and 'very tired' as they coped with the devastation of bombing. In cities some district nurses undertook duty in rest centres assisting people who had been bombed, and many went visiting patients, giving treatment and delivering babies in conditions of great danger with unexploded bombs all around. At the end of the war Lord Athlone sent a message to all Queen's nurses: 'You performed a national service by remaining at your posts. . . . I commend you all for your steadfast service so quietly and cheerfully carried out and for your courage so often unsung'.[4]

During the war the government had been forced to play a greater role in providing care for those whom the national emergency had deprived of services, and in 1941, a Committee of Reconstruction was set up to plan for after the war. In 1942, Sir William Beveridge presented his Report on Social Insurance and Allied Services which showed that a comprehensive service for the prevention and cure of disease and the restoration of the capacity for work should be available to all members of the community. Beveridge envisaged that his proposed legislation would be sufficient to lay the five giants of squalor, ignorance, idleness, want, and disease. The ensuing legislation had a profound effect on the work of the district nurse, and also had very considerable consequences for the Institute.

THE NATIONAL HEALTH ACT 1946

The most controversial part of the plan, and the most debated, was the National Health Act of 1946, debates which the Institute watched with keen interest. The Act set out to give a comprehensive medical service to all, but because of the opposition of doctors and the conflict of interest between the powerful voluntary hospital lobby and the equally powerful local authority lobby, the end result was the fixing of the services as they had developed so far in a tripartite structure with the cracks thinly papered over. The curative, preventive and the general practitioner services were divorced from one another, and there was little provision for liaison or communication; this failure would have a profound effect on the work of district nurses, and would result in them being wrongly used and undervalued.

Community health services, previously administered by the counties and county boroughs, became the local authority services as defined in Part III of the Act and known as LHAs. Apart from the whole range of maternity and child welfare services, the local authorities were to provide 'domiciliary and midwifery services and engage in activities for the prevention of illness and the care and after care of persons who were sick or physically disabled'.[5] Before the Act many local authorities worked through agencies such as the Queen's Institute and the Ranyard Mission, and the former was hopeful that this state of affairs would continue. After the Act the LHAs were the employers of district nurses paying them on the new Rushcliffe Scale, and then later on the scales laid down by the Nurses and Midwives Whitley Council.

In 1947, before the Act came into force, there were negotiations between the County Council Associations, the Association of Municipal Corporations and the Queen's Institute which: 'Led to arrangements whereby the LHAs providing a district nursing service are enabled to enter into direct membership with the Institute, an arrangement similar to the affiliation of voluntary committees'.[6] At the same time the Ministry of Health made it clear to the Institute that the headquarter's expenditure in connection with the Queen's training of nurses must be regarded as part of the general expenditure of the Institute.

REDEFINING THE COUNCIL'S WORK

The Council of the Institute now redefined its work as follows:

(1) To recruit SRNs for work in the domiciliary field as district nurses, district nurse midwives and district health visitors.

(2) To organise the district training of such nurses in homes approved by the Institute through the goodwill of the LHAs and the nursing associations to whom the homes belong.

(3) To provide courses for SEANs.

(4) Through its officers to pay periodic visits to those areas where Queen's nurses are employed and generally to act in an advisory capacity.

(5) To keep a Roll of Queen's nurses.

(6) To organise refresher courses, each course being approved by the Ministry of Health.

(7) To arrange conferences on subjects pertaining to district nurses.

(8) To organise health visitor training centres at Brighton and Bolton combined with district nursing.

(9) To answer queries and give practical assistance to applications from the dominions, colonies and foreign countries.

(10) To administer a number of trust funds for the benefit of persons connected with, or allied to, the district nursing service.

The district nursing associations now shed the irksome task of trying to find money to pay the salaries of district nurses, but they still had a role to play in the running of the homes. In order to retain voluntary status the district nursing associations continued to provide a percentage of the total running costs of the service. This practice continued until rising salaries and the changed public attitude towards the provision of services made this an anachronism. However, even after they ceased to provide financial support a number of associations remained active in the cause of district nursing.

During the war there had been discussions with the Ministry about postwar plans for district nursing, though at that stage it was by no means sure what form the National Health Service would take. The Ministry was not in agreement with giving the control of training to the Queen's Institute, because there were other organisations involved and because there were only 4476 Queen's nurses out of some 9203 practising district nurses. However, it was generally agreed that a common standard of training was necessary and that the training should be controlled by a central committee. The Royal College of Nursing (the 'Royal' was added in 1939), with its Public Health Section, was also concerned in the negotiations, and agreed to a common training but did not agree to the Queen's Institute being the examining body.[7] The College had just published the Horder Report advocating a basic nurse training which included social medicine and an elective six months in a speciality in the last year of training. There were, it claimed, already too many examining bodies which was confusing to the profession and to the public. The College hoped that such courses would all eventually be controlled by the profession itself under the aegis of the General Nursing Council, a hope that had to await the demise of the General Nursing Council and nearly 40 years of campaigning before it came about.

In 1947 the situation was further complicated by the fact that the government had set up its own working party on the Recruitment and Training of Nurses under the chairmanship of Sir Robert Wood, and the Minister of Health, Iain Macleod, decided to wait for its recommendations before making any decision on district nurse training. The air was full of excuses for doing nothing. The Institute's case was weakened by the fact that by no means all the LHAs looked to them for advice and training; 56 authorities used voluntary agencies which included the Queen's Institute, thirteen had a mixed system, and no less than 60 provided their own nursing service. Half the district nurses who were employed had no training, and not all the authorities thought it necessary. The situation was exacerbated by the question of pay. In 1948, when the Whitley Councils were set up, the Queen's Institute applied for a place on the staff side to represent district nurses, but the claim was turned down because it represented too few nurses and it had not been a negotiating body before. The decision was not surprising in view of the already unwieldy nature of the staff side, but it was a blow to the Institute in its claim to being the mouthpiece of district nurses.

EARLY DAYS OF THE NHS

In the meantime the NHS was treating a backlog of cases, and in order to do so it was putting a premium on early discharge from hospital. New technology and drugs revolutionised medicine, and as more cases became treatable and curable the work of the district nurse changed and her burden increased. Contrary to the service before the war, many district nurses were now married, and in 1947 the Queen's Institute recruited its first male nurse. Now nurses were often less willing, and less able, to go away to a centre for six months' training, especially if the employing authority did not seem to think it necessary. All these factors made the Institute's position more difficult.

District nurse training

In 1953 the Ministry of Health discussed the concept of the 'domiciliary team' and this again raised the question of district nurse training. By now it was obvious that there was going to be little action on the Wood report, and that there would be no radical change in the basic nurse training. There was now diversity of district nurse trainings and no training. In order to rationalise the situation the Ministry of Health set up a working party under the chairmanship of Sir Frederick Armer, a deputy secretary at the Ministry of Health. The working party consisted of five Ministry officials, four LHA representatives, five medical officers and three nurses, two of whom were district nurses. The composition of the working party was in itself an indication of the attitude of the Ministry of Health to district nursing. It was also an indication of the lack of political power on the part of the nursing profession at that time.

A number of organisations gave evidence, of which the Queen's Institute was the most important. It had 55 training centres and trained some 700 district nurses a year in courses lasting six months for nurses with district experience, and four months for health visitors, mid-wives and nurses with 18 months' district experience. Miss Merry, the General Superintendent, and Dr Struthers, who represented medical officers of health on the Council of the Institute, gave evidence. They refuted the argument that the length of training was a deterrent to nurses wanting to be district nurses, and attributed the lack of candidates to the poor pay and long hours. They outlined the wide variety of tasks now undertaken by the district nurse, and urged most strongly that the course should be compulsory, that it should last at least six months and that the Queen's Institute should become the national central body.[8]

The Royal College of Nursing, in its evidence, did not necessarily support the plea for six months, arguing that the trend was towards shorter training; it felt there should be fewer centres, preferably in universities or centres of higher education, with the students supernumerary to the service needs of the district, and with the fieldwork controlled by the training institute. The clash of views about the length of training was largely due to the pious hope that existed at that time that the basic training course would be more comprehensive. In the event the Queen's Institute took the more realistic view. The College's plan, eventually put into practice nearly 30 years later, was too ambitious at that time. On the other hand, the Ranyard Mission supported the Queen's Institute in its plea for a six-month training period. The real difficulty lay with the LHAs who were determined that the course, when it came, would be shorter and cheaper — the cheaper the better.

In view of the evidence against it the Institute reviewed its position, but after consideration it felt that it could not agree to a training of less than six or four months, though it did agree to some flexibility. In order to support its case the Institute took expert opinion from professors of education who examined the Institute's syllabus to see if it could be taken in a shorter period; the unanimous decision was that it could not. Indeed, Professor Lauwery, Professor of Comparative Education at the University of London, thought that it should be longer.[9] Armed with this evidence, the Institute reapproached the working party, but to no avail. Minds were made up. What was uppermost in the minds of the Ministry officials was the rising cost of the health service. The Ministry made it clear that they did not want a minority report and hinted darkly that the Institute would suffer if it refused to concede to a shortened course. If it did agree to the four or three month formula then it would be possible for the LHAs to continue to use the Institute for training.

During 1956 the Education Committee of the Institute prepared a syllabus to cover a five-month course with more student status which it hoped would be an acceptable compromise. However, it was rejected by the Institute's Education Committee which now reverted to its stand on the six-month course. Miss Merry and Dr Struthers were now advised to prepare a minority report which they did, and to which they attached their expert reports. These the working party refused to accept, and there was what Miss Merry described as 'some unpleasantness', which was probably a masterpiece of understatement. The Institute had been battering against a closed door.

In October 1956 the Minister of Health, Robin Turton, addressed the annual meeting of the Queen's Institute at Church House, Westminster and told them that he had decided to accept the Armer Report. A four or three month training course would be laid down as a minimum standard and authorities could opt for a longer course if they wished. The Minister was coolly received. Mr Wedderburn, the Vice-Chairman of the Queen's Institute, summed up the feelings of the meeting in his vote of thanks.

He [the Minister] has sounded the death knell of one of the most cherished ideals of the Queen's Institute. . . . Our earnest hope was that as in all other branches of the Public Health Service there should be officially recognised a single and high national qualification for district nurses.[10]

Mr Wedderburn was undoubtedly thinking of the unfortunate comparison that would be drawn between the academic qualifications of the district nurse and the health visitor, and events were to show that Mr Wedderburn was cast that day in the role of Cassandra.

The Armer report discussed the different responsibilities of district nurses and the difficulties they faced working on their own, but it argued that the need for training was now affected by the new syllabus of the GNC which was more comprehensive and gave the general nurse an insight into the needs of the community. This as it turned out was a piece of wishful thinking. However, the most damning part of the report was the fact that it considered that there was no need for a statutory body to control training. A central body was to be set up to issue a syllabus and a national certificate, and the LHAs and the Queen's Institute should be responsible for training.[11]

The minority report was published and the debate continued in the nursing press. The Institute argued that the new GNC syllabus would make little difference to the orientation of new candidates who would need as much adjustment to their lifestyle as before, and that the shorter training would lower the prestige of district nurses in the eyes of their colleagues,[12] a forecast that was, unfortunately, to prove correct.

One of the outcomes of the Armer report was the fact that the LHAs who did not use the Queen's Institute tended to group their district nurses for surveillance under their medical officer of health. Comparatively few appointed a district nursing superintendent. Instead, control was often delegated to an assistant medical officer, which meant that district nurses were accountable to an officer of another discipline. The Queen's Inspectors may have been unduly particular about cupboards, books and bags but, as their reports show, they were sensitive enough to change nurses when there were personality difficulties; now often there was no one to whom the district nurse could turn, an anomaly that was not put right until the Mayston report of 1968.

In spite of its disappointments in its battle with the Ministry of Health the Queen's Institute now turned its attention to improving the education of district nurses by other means. The Nurses Act 1949 encouraged experimentation and officers of the Queen's Institute engaged in teaching and examining district nurses were convinced that the existing training of district nurses did not fit them for the comprehensive health care expected from a National Health Service and rising expectations. In 1957 an experiment with eleven students was set up between Hammersmith Hospital, the Queen's Institute and Battersea College (later the University of Surrey) in which selected students covered the syllabuses of the General Nursing Council, Part 1 certificate of the Central Midwives Board, the Royal Society for the Promotion of Health, and the Queen's Institute. Every effort was made to prevent unnecessary overlapping on the subject matter common to the four courses, and selected students had to have five subjects with the General Certificate of Education, two of which were at A level. The course attracted a high level of candidates, and when it was assessed some ten years later it was shown that the students had a lower dropout rate than in traditional courses and, interestingly enough, most applied to work in the public health field.[13] Here was proof, if proof were needed, that candidates were not put off by a more academic course, that there was much overlapping in the different courses, and that such integrated courses attracted students who might otherwise be lost to the profession. It was a vindication of the Institute's argument.

In 1950 the Queen's Institute was also the innovator of the combined courses started at the Bolton Technical College and at the Art and Social Studies Department of the Brighton Technical College which enabled suitable candidates to take the Queen's Institute District Nurse Course with the Health Visitor course in a shorter period. Again both courses attracted a higher standard of candidates and tended to be oversubscribed.

Change was in the air. Experiments showed that, given better selection, candidates were capable of taking composite courses that avoided overlapping in a shorter period and that the end product was as efficient as the traditional system. From the viewpoint of the Queen's Institute and health visiting, the disadvantage of the traditional system was the fact that the basic nurse training course was heavily hospital- and task-orientated, and until this was changed it was not possible to prepare a nurse for work in the community in a shorter time. Everything depended on the foundation block. But the profession was not united; the pages of the nursing press were filled with calls for shorter training, or, conversely, a long comprehensive training — for, on the one hand, a single portal of entry, on the other, a two-tier system. Matrons were foraging overseas for pairs of hands for the service needs of hospitals, and were fearful that better selection would mean fewer nurses. The British Medical Association was at least united; it was against the higher education and better selection of student nurses; nurses were there to do the doctor's bidding. Overall there was the attitude of the government. Alarmed by the rising cost of the health service, the government was looking for a nurse training that was shorter and preferably cheaper, and post-basic training was not a priority.

This was a difficult period for the Council of the Institute now under the chairmanship of the Dowager Lady Rayleigh, well-known for her efforts on the part of district nurses in Essex, and ably supported by Mr Wedderburn, the chairman of the Executive Council which bore the brunt of the difficult negotiations with the Ministry of Health. There were a number of reasons why the Council failed to achieve its objective of becoming the accepted training body and the mouthpiece for district nurses. Nurses are notoriously factious, not all district nurses supported the Queen's Institute, some saw it as an elitist body. There were other organisations representing district nurses and indeed, trade unions. This was the period when it was believed that once the backlog of disease was treated, ill-health would wither away; the government had yet to learn that good care creates a further need for care. It was also forecast that the high rate of marriage would reduce the need for professional carers in the home, a forecast that on a number of counts was to prove wrong. The whole attitude both in the civil service and in the hospitals was that no specialist skills were required to nurse patients at home. Moreover, in the early days of the service, in this brave new world of state medicine, the Ministry saw a voluntary organisation like the Queen's Institute as an irritation and an anachronism.

In spite of these setbacks and its difficult postwar situation the Institute did not give up, it continued to provide refresher courses and a wide variety of services, including films and a library for nurses; it started an overseas fund and continued providing district nurse training throughout Great Britain for the authorities with which it had an agreement. That it did so was a testimony to the value placed on its training by the profession itself. To be a Queen's nurse was the hallmark of professional excellence in a district nurse.

NOTES

1. *Queen's Nurses' Magazine*, editorial, September 1939, p. 312.
2. Queen's Institute of District Nursing Annual Report 1944, p. 8.
3. Women's Group on Public Welfare, *Our Towns*, Oxford University Press, Oxford, 1943.
4. Wilmshurst, M., *Record of the Work of the Queen's Nurses during*

the Second World War, pp. 7 and 15, Queen's Institute of District Nursing, 1945.

5. The National Health Service Act 1946, Part III, HMSO, London.

6. The Queen's Institute of District Nursing Annual Report 1963 (summarising the history of the Institute since the Act).

·7. The Royal College of Nursing Council Minutes, October 1946.

8. The Queen's Institute of District Nursing Council Minutes, February 1954.

9. White, R., *The Effects of the NHS on the Nursing Profession 1948-1961*, King's Fund, London, 1985, p. 151.

10. *Queen's Nurses' Magazine* January 1957, pp. 5-10.

11. The Queen's Institute of District Nursing Annual Report, 1956.

12. Black, A., The training of the district nurse, *Nursing Times*, 16 September 1955, 1031.

13. Bryden, E.G.M., *Integrated Course of Nurse Education — A Study of an Experiment*, Queen's Institute of District Nursing, 1969.

9

Postwar Policies for District Nursing

The acceptance of the Armer report by the Ministry was a blow to the Queen's Institute and a loss to district nursing in general, the official arguments seeming to imply that with changed health needs and a different basic nurse training, district nurses would need little preparation. The next quarter of a century of the Institute's life was spent in trying to mitigate the harm done and to restore district nursing to the primacy it once had.

First, it issued a new syllabus and encouraged as many health authorities as possible to use it, and of the 145 authorities no less than 121 were affiliated to the Institute and paid an annual subscription.[1] In 1957, when the District Nursing Advisory Committee was set up under the chairmanship of D.H. Ingall at the Ministry of Health, this time, out of a committee of twelve, four were Queen's nurses, with Miss Dora Williams, the Superintendent of Home Nursing in Plymouth, representing the Institute.[2] The Ingall committee had to work within the confines of the Armer report, but its recommendations did bring some improvements within the system that the Institute had been forced to accept *faute de mieux*. There was to be a National Committee for District Nursing with a panel of assessors to advise the Minister who would examine schemes for training, and there was to be a National Certificate for successful candidates. It was agreed that Ministry of Health nursing officers should make a periodic inspection of the training courses and that they would hold practical and oral examinations. The panel of assessors, chosen by the Advisory Committee, was set up in 1959, but contrary to the high hopes it was soon found that the panel had little power; the assessors became absorbed into a departmental committee of the civil service and were a training body without professional staff. In vain the panel protested vociferously about their lack of facilities but their pleas were ignored.

The panel had no power except to set an examination and to issue the National Certificate which was signed by the chief nursing officers of the different counties. At local level the courses and training facilities were largely unsupervised; candidates protested that they were of little value and that the National Certificate was not worth the paper it was written on. The response of the Institute was to arrange new schemes of training itself, modifying the length but affording more student status, and as a result its recruitment stayed at a satisfactory level. The Institute now regarded the National Certificate as of little consequence, and they continued to press for a national course of a higher standard to be made mandatory.

THE JAMESON REPORT

In 1956, before the Ingall committee on district nurse training had been set up, the working party under the chairmanship of Sir Wilson Jameson on the training and education of health visitors had reported. This had consequences for district nurses and unwittingly widened the gap between the two disciplines. The Jameson committee suggested that the role of the health visitor should be wider than that suggested by the Act:

> the health visitor should be a common point of reference and a source of standard information, a common advisor on health teaching, a common factor in the family welfare . . . she should be in a real sense a general purpose family visitor.[3]

The report recommended that the foundation for the health visitor's course should be the possession of the School Certificate, the registered nurse's training and obstetric experience, and that the course itself should involve greater study in social and mental health and should be linked with universities.[3] The nursing profession itself at that time did not ask for the possession of the School Certificate with five subjects as a condition of entry, therefore not all registered nurses could be health visitors, and this led to certain feelings of superiority which sometimes had an unfortunate effect on the harmony of the primary care team.

The Queen's Institute, while welcoming much of the Jameson report, had its reservations.[4] The Institute deprecated the emphasis put on the health visitor undertaking aftercare and rehabilitation in conjunction with general practitioners. This it saw as a duplication of the work of the district nurse, and it was feared that the health visitor would call in the district nurse 'which is quite unacceptable to district nurses and which can only lead to bad relationships instead of mutual confidence', a comment that recalls articles in the *Queen's Nurses' Magazine* some 40 years earlier. However, the real criticism came over the question of combined work. The Jameson report did not recommend combined work as a general principle, but did 'not see grounds for altering arrangements in areas where combined work existed'. The Institute was quick to point out that combined work was carried out in eighteen counties and that the system 'was economical and popular with staff and clients alike'. The other point of contention was the comment in the Jameson report that in future: 'health visitors will not be practising nurses and home nurses will not be highly trained health educators and social advisers', a point with which the civil service was no doubt delighted to agree when planning the training of the district nurse, but which the Institute deprecated. It smacked of belittling the district nurse and it looked like arrogance.

The dispute of half a century raised its head again. There is no doubt that during this period when many district nurses had no training, and health visitors were about to embark on a more heuristic course in an institute of higher education, that the difference rankled. Health visitors themselves, sometimes being compared unfavourably with social workers, were at times oversensitive and insecure about their own status and may have been tactless. The district nurses, on the other hand, often ignored by their colleagues in hospital, felt themselves lowly regarded, and they now saw themselves as being considered as second class nurses in the primary care team. It did not make for harmony in a team where so often the doctors did not understand either the work and capabilities of the district nurse, or the potential of the health visitor.

ATTACHMENT SCHEMES

The Jameson report suggested that health visitors work more closely with family practitioners; in 1956 the Guillebaud committee[5] which had been set up to look at the workings of the Health Service discussed arguments for integrating the hospital and community service. Integration was in the air, and there were to be many variations on the theme in the next few years. In 1955 two local authorities, Hampshire and Oxford City, decided to experiment by attaching health visitors to a selected group of general practitioners, an experiment watched with interest by the Queen's Institute and the Public Health Section of the Royal College of Nursing. The health visitors continued with their prime function, that of health education, but instead of working in a geographical area they were attached to group practices and covered families on the practice list. The experiments were encouraging. The general practitioners became more aware of the preventive aspect of medicine, and of the families of the patients on their list as opposed to the cases of the individuals who came to see them. Health visitors found their work more satisfying and less isolated, and although there were problems of adjustment, it was felt that the experiments should be adjusted to include district nurses and domiciliary midwives. Historically, general practitioners had not always worked closely with district nurses, and research was soon to show that the district nurse's abilities and potential were under-used.[6]

THE GILLIE COMMITTEE

In 1961 the Standing Medical Advisory Committee set up a subcommittee to study the future of general practice under the chairmanship of Dr (later Dame) Annis Gillie.[7] The committee found that general practitioners handled most medical episodes themselves without referring to any other agency, and that old people formed an increasing proportion of the population and took up more of the doctor's time, but all too often patients were isolated from their families and were unaware of the available facilities and how to obtain them. The committee came to the conclusion that greater cooperation between health and social workers was more important than changing the structure of the health service and they recommended that health visitors, district nurses and domiciliary midwives should, as far as possible, be attached to group practices.

The Queen's Institute welcomed the report and invited Dr Gillie to address their annual meeting. In 1963 experimental schemes were started and in the evaluation it was generally agreed that the health services were better used, communications improved, district nurses were treating more acutely ill patients, hospital admissions were saved and patients could be discharged earlier. Experiments spread and were generally accepted by district nurses, though there were losses as well as gains. There was a break with a long tradition of the nurse being responsible for her 'district' and some regretted the loss of a definable area where they were guide, philosopher and friend to the district and known to all. Furthermore, in some cases attachment was merely perfunctory; conversion to cooperation did not come to all doctors and nurses like the light on the Damascus Road. There is no doubt, however, that group attachment gradually changed the work of district nurses and was a watershed in their history. It changed the orientation of their work, and in some cases their duties and functions and it came, ironically, at a time when the status of district nurse training was at a low ebb.

THE LIVERPOOL CONNECTION

As the demands on district nurses changed, so the Queen's Institute tried to meet these needs with conferences, seminars, refresher courses and teaching material including educational films. In 1959, the Institute, looking back on 100 years of district nursing since William Rathbone started his scheme in Liverpool, decided to commemorate the occasion by launching a centenary appeal. The object of the appeal was to wipe out the deficit in the funds of £8 262, to provide money for the Institute's increasing overseas work (see Chapter 10) to enable the Institute to buy the lease of its headquarters at 57 Lower Belgrave Street and thereby eliminate the overhead costs, and to launch the William Rathbone Staff College. The appeal, which involved much hard work on the part of Queen's nurses themselves, raised the splendid sum of £201 358.

With the growing needs of the National Health Service, it had long been realised that nurses needed an opportunity to train for administration. The achievement of this aim was made possible by the generosity of the Liverpool Queen Victoria Nursing Association in handing over their Central Nurses' Home to the Queen's Institute for the nation, fully furnished and equipped to be 'the first residential Staff College for administrators and lecturers in the field of district nursing in this country and abroad'.[8]

In October 1960 the William Rathbone Staff College was opened by Princess Alice, Countess of Athlone, herself a granddaughter of Queen Victoria, the founder of the Institute. In this centenary year it was appropriate that the new College should be sited in Liverpool in the name of the founding father of trained district nurses. The College opened its doors to students in 1960 and continued to arrange residential and non-residential courses that were much appreciated both at home and overseas by students of various nursing disciplines. The College stayed open until 1975 when the Institute's deficit had risen to the alarming figure of £45 867 and it was decided that this valued, but expensive, establishment could no longer be afforded, and a working party was set up to arrange the winding up of the educational work and the ultimate sale of the premises. Apart from inflation, a main reason for the College not paying its way was the fact that not enough LHAs sent candidates to Liverpool, and after the Senior Management Structure report a duty was laid on the health service itself to provide management courses at all levels; other organisations and consultancy firms rushed in — management training was a growth industry. Finally, in 1974, with the reorganisation of the health service, there were fewer candidates. With the benefit of hindsight, and for the good of the financial health of the Institute, it might have been better if the College had been closed earlier, but at the time the Council was obviously reluctant to abandon its pioneering project and to sever its links with Liverpool.

THE MAYSTON REPORT

The needs for management training had come about due to the attempts to rationalise the structure of senior nursing posts both in hospital and in the community. In the community health service local government had developed its own hierarchy into which doctors and nurses had to be fitted; this pattern was varied and there was often confusion about the chain of command and the channels of communication. In 1968 a working party was set up under the chairmanship of Edward Mayston to advise on senior nursing posts in the community, taking into account the current, but not agreed, proposals for the unification of the health service and the growing practice of group attachment. The report recommended that the structure for senior nursing posts in the community be based on geography: at the top there should be chief nursing officers; and below area and senior nursing officers with each arm of the service having its own line of accountability. The report was good news for district nurses because it recognised their independent status and provided them with a senior nursing officer with experience in district nursing. The Queen's Institute welcomed the report and cooperated in organising management courses to meet the new needs.[9]

117

REORGANISATION OF 1974

The ink was barely dry on the Mayston report when the first discussion document on the reorganisation of the health service was put out. Documents followed in quick succession, each one having potential consequences for district nursing. In 1974, after a change of government, there was a change of plan, and Sir Keith Joseph introduced his management arrangements in a reorganised health service.[10] In order to unify the services, the *raison d'être* of the exercise, a cumbersome structure was introduced with regional and area health authorities as employing authorities. The post of medical officer of health was abolished and the community health services, but not the family practitioner committees, came under the area health authority, who at district level, may, or may not, have had a community care division.[10] This change of employing authority was a source of trauma to district nurses many of whom, with some justification, did not understand the new strucure, nor often did the doctors with whom they worked. Before they had come to terms with being employed by an area health authority the service was again reorganised and districts became the employing authority. All this was happening when district nurse training was at a low ebb, and although the Queen's Institute continued to put on conferences, courses and seminars it could not meet all the needs.

RESEARCH

One need that was paramount in the 1960s was that of research. The Institute's brushes with the Ministry of Health had shown how little they, and their advisers, had understood the value of a district nursing service, the vital role it could play in the economy of the health service and the damage the lack of such a service could do in terms of human suffering. In 1963, a gift of £15 000 for three years from the Miriam Marks Charitable Trust enabled the Council to set up a Research Department. Miriam, Lady Marks was for many years a member of the Institute's Council, and was an active worker and benefactor in the cause of district nursing and the Council was delighted at being able to pursue research 'in a more scientific manner'. Miss Lisbeth Hockey was appointed as Nursing Research Officer and the first project 'to explore the extent to which the district nursing service might be improved by the use of pre-sterilised equipment' was published in 1965.[11] But the Research Department will be mainly remembered for two publications which influenced the growth of primary care teams and the unification of the health service, one of which a Minister of Health declared he carried around with him. *Feeling the Pulse*, published in 1966 (see note 6) was a study designed to gather information on which to base the training and education of the district nurse. The study showed that district nurses were not being used to their potential, a high proportion of their time was spent on travelling and clerical duties, they were distracted by non-nursing duties and general practitioners were often ignorant of their qualifications. Patients needing treatment were either sent to hospital or were dealt with by doctors, and district nurses were confined to the care of the elderly. The report concluded that district nurses were not fulfilling the role expected of them and that they could play a greater part in both nursing the patients at home and in helping doctors. The study, coming as it did in the wake of the Gillie report, helped to stimulate attachment schemes and bring an awareness that the primary care team could meet more of the health needs of the population.

Care in the Balance,[12] published two years later, had if anything a greater impact, for it showed cost-conscious secretaries of state that the increasingly expensive hospital service was being used wastefully. The survey was designed to test the hypothesis that patients were discharged from hospital without having the full range of domiciliary services made available to them, and that patients attended outpatients' departments for treatment that could be given at home. From the data collected and analysed the research team came to the conclusion that a high proportion of patients were discharged to the outpatients' department as a matter of routine and often returned to the wards for dressings that could be done at home. Many patients found these visits a source of anxiety and because of the rush of hospital routine and their tension they did not understand their instructions. As there was little or no communication with the community service, doctors and district nurses could do little to help. The second part of the survey showed that there was a vast area of unmet need; few patients knew their entitlements, and how they got their dressings and other medical needs was largely a matter of chance. Again there was ignorance about the qualifications of the district nurse, ignorance that reflected the limitations of the basic training for both doctors and nurses.

These reports and others like *Home from Hospital*[13] demonstrate the validity of the Institute's case in its stand for a higher training for district nurses and a qualification that was recognised nationally. By the time *Care in the Balance* was published it was realised that ill-health would not wither away and that there would be a rising demand for care in the community. The National Health Service had been hospital-orientated, the corridors of power at the Ministry were trodden by the upper echelons from the hospital world. Now, rather late, it was realised that the future might lie in a world elsewhere from hospitals and high technology. The Queen's Institute tried to make its voice heard, but it had been hampered by its voluntary status, the lack of data and research-based evidence with which to back its case, the attitude of hospital matrons and, above all, the attitude of general practitioners, who were obsessed by the need to preserve their status as independent practitioners with a contract *for* service. Not until their surgeries were overwhelmed did they see the value of a primary care team. It is this interlude, before the light dawned, that gave the Queen's Institute its most difficult years. Unable to influence the priorities of the health service they were pushed back to meeting immediate short-term needs, and for two decades they reacted to events as they happened and tried to provide services to meet each change. This in the long run was to overwhelm their resources.

NOTES

1. *Queen's Nurses' Magazine*, September 1957, p. 130.
2. Queen's Institute of District Nursing Annual Report, 1957.
3. Ministry of Health, *An Inquiry into Health Visiting*, Report of the Working Party, 1956; and summary of recommendations.
4. *Queen's Nurses' Magazine*, June 1957, pp. 88–9.
5. Ministry of Health, *Report on the Committee of Enquiry into the Costing of the National Health Service*, Cmnd 9663. HMSO, London.
6. Hockey, L., *Feeling the Pulse*, Queen's Institute of District Nursing, 1966.
7. Ministry of Health, *Future Scope of General Practice*, HMSO, London, 1963.
8. *Liverpool Daily Post*, 7 October 1960.
9. Queen's Institute of District Nursing Annual Report, 1970, p. 11.
10. *Management Arrangements in the Reorganised National Health Service*, London, HMSO, 1972. (Hospital and Community Nursing Divisions.)
11. *Safer Sterilizing of Equipment: A study of traditional methods of sterilizing in current district nursing practice in selected areas, and of the provisions of pre-sterilized supplies for the domiciliary health team by local authorities throughout England and Wales*, Queen's Institute of District Nursing, 1965.
12. Hockey, L., *Care in the Balance*, Queen's Institute of District Nursing, 1968.
13. Skeet, M., *Home from Hospital*, Dan Mason Research, Macmillan, London, 1970.

10

The Old Order Changeth

By an irony of fate, during the postwar years while the Queen's Institute was fighting its battle with the Ministry to represent district nurses and to become a national training body, its influence overseas was increasing. From its earliest days the Institute had been interested in spreading a system of district nursing abroad. In 1898, with the aid of the Council, Lady Aberdeen had started the Victorian Order of Nurses in Canada, while in 1896, Mr Boulton, Secretary of the Queen's Commemoration Fund, had put forward an ambitious plan for federating district nursing institutions overseas with the Queen's Institute in London. In the first half of the century visitors, both lay and professional, came to the Institute for advice, one of the most important being Mrs Mary Breckinridge who, in 1924, came to the Institute to study district nursing in Britain before starting her Frontier Service of nurses on horseback in Kentucky.

NURSING IN THE DEVELOPING COUNTRIES

It was, however, in the postwar period when the needs of the developing countries became paramount that the Queen's Institute played its most important role in overseas nursing. In 1946, immediately after the war, the Greek War Relief Association arranged for a group of 50 students from Greece to come to Great Britain under the care of Miss Merry, who was then the Education Officer at the Institute, to train as general, midwifery and district nurses in five years. This was an ambitious undertaking, and not without its trauma, as the Greek girls expected student status and not the British apprenticeship system where they worked as they learned. However, in spite of the high marriage rate, homesickness and the conflict about working in hospitals, 23 completed their course and returned to Greece, a triumph for the tact and patience of the Institute's nursing officers.[1]

Malta

The same year, with the help of Lady Lacock, the wife of the Governor of Malta, the Malta District Nursing Association was founded and six Queen's nurses under Miss Grazier, a Queen's Superintendent, set up an embryo district nursing service for the island. For the next 20 years the Institute sent out nurses, provided a tropical uniform, sent out superintendents to advise and the Chief Nursing Officer to make a triennial visit. It was a two-way traffic; Maltese nurses came to England to be trained while relays of Queen's nurses went to Malta to help organise, to impress on the government the need for such a service and to sort out the religious difficulties. Finally, in 1968, Miss Jefferies and her two remaining British nurses returned home, it being the intention of the Memorial Association to employ all Maltese nurses in the future. The torch had been handed on. The Queen's Institute had played an important role in the development of the island's health and social services in the troubled political climate in Malta after the war and it says much for the skill and patience of the Queen's nurses that British participation lasted so long.

Back home the Institute was receiving ever more calls for advice from overseas. Like Britain, most countries were reorganising their health services and placing more emphasis on community care. Visitors came, not only from the developing countries, but from former dominions, the United States, Israel, Poland, Chile, the Scandinavian countries, and there were contacts with the World Health Organisation.

Jamaica

In 1957 the Hyacinth Lightbourne Visiting Service was inaugurated in Jamaica with the aid of the Queen's Institute Overseas Fund and Miss Rosalie Hunt, a Queen's nurse, was seconded for six months to pioneer district nursing services in Jamaica; later the project was helped by the Nuffield Trust. The following year a Queen's trained nurse was appointed to Christiana. For the next ten years the Institute was closely associated with the district nursing service in Jamaica, which, like Malta, became affiliated with the Queen's Institute in

England, and in spite of the successive economic crises to which that island was prone, the scheme spread and played an important part in Jamaica's health services.

PRIMARY CARE IN AFRICA

The need for primary health care in Africa had been long recognised, but after the war, with increasing populations, the need was more urgent. In 1957, Lady Twining, the wife of the Governor of Tanganyika, visited the Institute to discuss the development of a district nursing service in that country. A scheme was drawn up and the Institute sent out Miss Amy Large to pioneer the work. The following year Miss Charlotte Kratz took over the difficult task of organising a service for a population composed of many different races and creeds where the need for health education was urgent. In 1961, after negotiations conducted by Miss Dixon, the Deputy Superintendent of the Institute, the government of Tanganyika took over the service in a modified form and Miss Kratz became the Nursing Officer superintending the service, and for a number of years the Institute maintained close links with Tanganyika.

WORLDWIDE CONNECTIONS

During this period the Queen's Institute played an important role on the world stage. The General Superintendent, (later the CNO) Miss Joan Gray, was indefatigable in her travels; she not only paid triennial visits to the Institute's affiliates but visited services in the United States, Singapore, Yugoslavia, India, Hong Kong, Kuala Lumpur, Fiji and Labrador as well as spending periods in New Zealand and Australia. In 1969, before she retired, Miss Gray took on a heavy schedule of visiting organisations and governments all round the world. It was like a royal tour with four engagements a day in seventeen different parts of the world, a testimony to the influence of the Institute in the wider world.

Back home she and her nursing officers were receiving nurses, government officials and representatives from all parts of the world. Polish and Spanish nurses, midwives from Chile, gynaecologists from Trinidad, professors from Texas, and matrons from Canada, it was all grist to the Institute's mill, but it was, of course, a strain on the resources of the Institute, whose traditional base, voluntary contributions, was now eroded.[2]

Though there is still much to be done, as famine in Africa makes us all too well aware, nevertheless the standard of primary care throughout many parts of the world has improved since the Second World War. Much of this is due to an improved standard of living in a number of countries, but it is also due to better health education and the part played by the World Health Organisation and its agencies assisted by many voluntary organisations of which the Queen's Institute has been one.

CHANGES AT HOME

At home changes were taking place both at the Institute and in the local associations. The Queen's Institute had come into the National Health Service trailing the clouds of its former charitable status. Locally it had been run by district nursing associations, usually composed of distinguished citizens or landowners who raised money for 'their' nurses. As old Queen's nurses were apt to say, they were financed by 'jam and jumbles'. In Reading, the local association, celebrating its Jubilee in 1947, explained in its souvenir publication that 'their nurses', in spite of what some people thought, 'were hospital trained but they were also very human . . . take a peep into their bedrooms and you will find treasured photographs of relatives and friends, little vases of flowers, pots of powder and cream that find a place in every woman's room'.[3]

The Committee presumably inspected the bedrooms of 'their' nurses, which although probably kindly meant, seems today like excessive paternalism. The nurses, the writer pointed out, started their day with prayers before setting off on their bicycles on 'their mission to the sick'. It was an image that district nurses wanted to dispel, but in some places change came slowly. Not all associations, and certainly not all doctors, were convinced that the Health Service was a move in the right direction, and after 40 years it is difficult to recall the hostility it once engendered in some quarters. The local associations had raised the money for the district nursing service and for some years to come the aura of charity remained.

NURSING IN THE 1960s

The Council in London, nominated by its patron Queen Elizabeth, the

Queen Mother, consisted of distinguished people, many of whom like the Dowager Duchess of Richmond and Gordon, the Dowager Lady Rayleigh, Caroline, Viscountess Bridgeman, the Lady Brooke of Cumnor and Lady Heald had given years of devoted service to the Institute, and many of whom had been instrumental in raising money for funds before the National Health Service. They were the rock on which the Institute developed. But over the years the Council had become large and, apart from the Council, there was a wide range of representative members from various associations connected with the Institute and from the federations representing geographical areas. The work was done by the Executive Council, but that was still large and, interestingly enough, did not have a Queen's nurse as a member. There was a vast array of subcommittees, the most important of which was probably the Education Committee, but the whole structure was unwieldly and not representative of district nursing in the 1960s.

In 1967 the Council decided to revise its constitution.

It was felt that the rather large and unselective body that had evolved over the years was unlikely, in present-day circumstances, to attract young, able and almost certainly busy members of various professions whose membership is most desirable.[4]

Accordingly, it was decided to reduce the number of representatives from some bodies, to allow others to lapse and to reduce the number of subcommittees. The new Council which emerged was, in fact, still large; William Rathbone, the fourth generation of that family to serve the Council, became Chairman, with Lady Heald as Vice-Chairman and the Lady Brooke of Cumnor Chairman of the Executive Committee. It was this reformed Council, with its various advisory committees, that had to preside over the great changes that were to occur in the Institute in the next ten years.

The first unpalatable fact that new Council had to face was a deficit of £19 342. The Institute was trying to provide too many services, and of these the most costly was the financing of training centres and the running of the practical and oral examinations for the Queen's Certificate. To abandon this was a terrible decision; this, after all, was why the Institute had been founded, but in 1966 the Council came to the conclusion that its examination had become a duplication:

it is, moreover, expensive duplication, since the procedures associated with the award impose a considerable load upon both professional and administrative staff. The cessation of the certificate will save the former eighteen weeks of practical examination each year, time which can be devoted to other activities . . .[5]

The Institute justified its decision by reporting an improvement in the regional arrangements for the National Certificate, a hope perhaps not shared by its educational officers who complained about the low standard. The announcement that the Queen's Institute was to cease training came as a shock to district nurses and to the profession as a whole, most of whom did not understand the sequence of events or the financial situation. It meant that eventually there would be no Queen's nurses, and, with widespread dissatisfaction with the National Certificate, the cause of raising the status of district nursing seemed lost in England, Scotland and Northern Ireland.

In Eire the situation was different. Here there were still Jubilee nurses and the Lady Dudley Nursing Service which had been started in 1903. It so happened that in 1967 the Department of Health for Ireland reorganised its outdoor nursing service, and after some abortive consultation the Jubilee nurses were absorbed into the local government service. The Lady Dudley nurses continued until as late as 1971 when they were also absorbed.[6] In 1968, it looked to most district nurses as if the end of an era had come.

However, the Institute still had an important role to play. The Department of Health did not recognise state enrolled nurses for district training. The Institute was an advocate for the use of enrolled nurses in the team, and it continued to arrange courses of instruction for them of which an increasing number took advantage. Freed from the need to provide the basic course, the Council and officers were able to pay more attention to post-basic courses, experimental schemes, research and work overseas. In the meantime the Council watched with concern the whole spectrum of nurse training. In 1969 the Institute submitted evidence to the Committee on Nursing which had been set up under the chairmanship of Professor (later Lord) Asa Briggs to make recommendations for the future training and education of nurses.[7]

This committee was important because it was the first to plan for nursing within a unified health service and based on total care. The committee recommended a single portal of entry with all students taking a foundation course leading to a Certificate in Nursing. Some students would stop there, others would go on and take modules in greater depth and become registered nurses. Finally, the Certificate of Higher Education would replace all separate examination boards and this, of course, included the National Certificate for District

126

Nurse Training. A further recommendation was that the General Nursing Council should be replaced by the United Kingdom Central Council (UKCC) and with national boards responsible for all nursing education both basic and post-basic.

The Briggs report

The recommendations were on the whole favourably received by the profession and in 1971 Professor Briggs addressed the Annual Meeting of the Institute. At last district nurses saw a chance of achieving parity with other disciplines in post-basic education. But it was not to be. Training bodies to be replaced were fearful for their speciality, and health visitors lobbied and eventually got a separate training Council. This display of faction threw district nurses back on their anomalous position; theirs would still be regarded as a second class training. In 1975 the Queen's Institute made a strong protest to the Department of Health expressing its concern that a statutory body had not been included in the proposals for the training of district nurses. It appeared that a central committee was not to be set up and that the national boards were to be left to establish their own pattern. The Institute was not alone in its protest; other organisations and the district nurses themselves lobbied vigorously, and in 1979 eventually got their own District Nursing Joint Committee under the aegis of the Central Council for Nursing, Midwifery and Health Visiting (UKCC). In 1983, when the national boards replaced the training bodies that had previously been responsible for the training and education of nurses, midwives and health visitors, the committee became operative with Miss Barbara Robottom, a Queen's nurse, as the Principal Professional Officer.

The new curriculum

In the meantime, a new curriculum for district nurse training was hammered out based on new educational concepts, the nursing process, nursing models, the extended role of the district nurse and the correlation of theory and practice. The course, which was to take place in Colleges of Higher Education, was six months in duration with one-third of the time allocated to practical teaching and experience, and was more demanding than the training it had replaced. In 1983, not without protest from some authorities, the course was made mandatory. The announcement at the annual meeting of the Queen's Institute raised a cheer, 'the fight was o'er the battle done'; at last it was recognised that *all* district nurses needed a special and higher education. This is, of course, what Miss Nightingale had said just over 100 years ago. District nursing now entered on a new phase.

THE INSTITUTE'S PROBLEM YEARS

While negotiations about district nurse training were going on, the Institute was looking at its structure and its future aims and purposes. The committees were again streamlined, and there was a higher proportion of nurse members with community health experience on the Council and, in keeping with modern trends, a greater proportion of the Council's affairs was entrusted to its officers. A new system of membership was introduced, which it was hoped would raise more money; in 1973, a Supplemental Charter was granted and the Queen's Institute of District Nursing became the Queen's Nursing Institute, a title felt to be more in keeping with modern times and the contemporary pattern of the health services.[8]

Unfortunately, these changes did little to keep the wolf from the door. In 1975 there was a deficit of £35 006 and it at last became apparent that the Institute could not continue to live beyond its means indefinitely. As a first step towards balancing the books it was decided to close the William Rathbone Staff College, a measure that Council took with great reluctance and one that was much regretted but understood by those many hundreds of nurses who had benefited from attendance at the College over the years.

Despite this step, 1976 saw the deficit grow to £47 848 and early in that year Council agreed that the Institute's educational role could be better met by special conferences and the *Queen's Nursing Journal*, the publication which had replaced the *Queen's Nurses' Magazine* in 1957.[9] 'Cuts' in health service expenditure — that recurring phenomenon of recent years — meant that there were fewer applicants for the courses organised by the Institute and Council agreed that there was no alternative but to dispense with the service of its nursing officers who had been responsible for its educational work. This was another blow to district nurses — there had been nursing officers at headquarters to 'warn, comfort and command' since 1890 and now they were no more. Surely the Institute seemed to be folding its tents.

Also in 1976 it was decided to recruit a chief administrator with responsibility for reassessing the Institute's future role and making recommendations on how best this role could be carried out, given the financial constraints then obtaining. Mr Philip Starr, who had had experience both in industry and in the charitable field, was appointed and took up the post in September.

In 1977 there were more economies and retrenchment. For nineteen years the *Queen's Nursing Journal* had served the interests of district nurses by providing them with material that helped them to keep up to date in the changing world, but publishing is an expensive business, and in 1977 the Council 'with sadness' decided to cease publication and to rely on the good offices of the *Nursing Mirror* to devote a section to community nursing interests. Marian Stringer, who had been on the staff of the Institute for 27 years, seventeen of which were as editor of the *Queen's Nursing Journal*, transferred to the *Nursing Mirror* to watch the interests of district nurses there until that publication finally merged with the *Nursing Times*.

In order to put its finances on a sound footing the Council, under the chairmanship of Mrs James Bull, an educationalist, agreed to give up the services like the Library and Information Department that could be met by other organisations and to concentrate on the activities that the Institute with its experience was in a unique position to perform. The first thing necessary for the Institute to have any future at all, was to be out of the red, and by dint of stringent economy, good housekeeping and making better use of the premises in Lower Belgrave Street, a surplus of £36 941 was achieved in 1978, the highest in the history of the Institute.

For the Institute and the Council these were difficult years and it looked to the outside world as if the Queen's Institute was a spent force, but as the 1980s dawned, with a new training there were new opportunities for district nurses, and new needs to be met. These the Institute seized, doing what it could do best, pioneering. The phoenix rose again.

NOTES

1. Greek War Association, correspondence 1946–63.
2. Queen's Institute of District Nursing Annual Report, 1969.
3. *The Queen Victoria Institute Reading*, Jubilee 1897–1947, Nicholls and Co., Reading, 1947.
4. Queen's Institute of District Nursing Annual Report, 1967.
5. Queen's Institute of District Nursing Annual Report, 1966.
6. Crowley, M.F., *A Century of Service 1880–1980 The Story of Nursing in Ireland* (no publisher), p. 26.

7. DHSS, *Report of the Committee on Nursing* (Briggs), London, HMSO, Cmnd 5115.

8. Queen's Nursing Institute Annual Report, 1973.

9. Queen's Institute of District Nursing Annual Report, 1957.

11

The Queen's Nursing Institute Today

One of the remarkable features of the Queen's Institute during the last 100 years has been the outstanding calibre, continuity and devotion of its Council. Founded by the personal interest of Queen Victoria, it has never lacked for royal patrons both for England and Scotland. Today it is honoured to have Her Majesty Queen Elizabeth The Queen Mother as Patron, and Her Royal Highness Princess Alice, Duchess of Gloucester as the President of both the English Institute and the Scottish Branch, while other members of the royal family often grace its proceedings.

The founding father of trained district nursing, and the guiding hand behind the early constitution of the Institute, was undoubtedly William Rathbone, who was the first Vice-President and Honorary Secretary, and of whom Miss Nightingale wrote when he died he was 'one of God's best and greatest sons'. In 1891 William was joined on the Council by his niece, Rosalind Paget, who remained a member until 1946. On the death of her uncle in 1902, the Rathbone torch was handed on to his son William Gair Rathbone, who shouldered the burden of the family business and gave much time and energy to the Institute through the troubled times early in the century until his untimely death in 1919. Then Mr Rathbone's place on the Council was taken by his daughter, Elena, Mrs Bruce Richmond, later to become Lady Richmond. For over 40 years until 1962, Lady Richmond served the Council for many years as Honorary Secretary, taking an active interest in the work of district nurses up and down the country, showing, like her grandfather, a remarkable capacity for welcoming change. In 1941 Lady Richmond represented district nurses on the Rushcliffe Committee set up to examine the pay and conditions of nurses and was a strong advocate in their cause. In 1935 a fourth generation of Rathbones joined the Council, another William

Rathbone, who in 1968 became Chairman of Council and remained so until the reorganisation in 1971 when he became a Vice-President. Today, the fifth generation, William Rathbone junior, is the Vice-Chairman of the Council and a trustee, thus giving 100 years of Rathbone association with the Queen's Nursing Institute.

The original Provisional Council included a Mrs Theodore Acland, a member of the Acland family by marriage who had been associated with Miss Nightingale and the early nursing reforms. Mrs Acland served the Council for a number of years as did Reginald Brodie Dyke Acland. Today Mrs Martin Acland, a relation by marriage, is the Chairman of Council, and to whose enthusiasm much is owed for the current resurgence of the Institute.

Looking back over a hundred years of Council membership one is struck by the length of service given by some members: for example, the Dowager Duchess of Richmond and Gordon, 57 years; Sir Dyce Duckworth over 30 years; Mrs Minet 32 years; and by recurring family names. The duty to support the cause of district nursing was often handed from mother to daughter and from father to son; like Elena Rathbone, some families 'were born to district nursing'.

There has also been a remarkable continuity in the trustees of the Institute; from the outset the cause attracted the highest advisers. Lord Rothschild was appointed in 1908 and a Rothschild was a trustee until 1986, the family serving almost as long as the Rathbones. In recent years the Institute has had the invaluable advice of the Hon. Sir John Baring and, thanks to the wise investment policies of the trustees, the Institute has been able to recover from its lean years and to expand its activities.

Today the Council, with a maximum of 24 members, is small in comparison with the pre-1967 era and is composed of a balanced representation from district nursing, community medicine, social service, nursing education and the world of finance. Thus advice and guidance is readily available, and freely given, on the main activities of the Institute and on any financial considerations.

While not being a negotiating body, the Institute, with its long experience of the specific needs of district nurses and their particular problems, continues to represent nurses on governmental and non-governmental bodies. Untrammelled by political connections and professional pressure the Institute is able to offer an objective viewpoint. To this end the Council is in close contact with the United Kingdom Central Council, the national boards and particularly with the District Nursing Joint Committee. Indeed, the contact was for a short time geographical as the Institute provided the Central Council with its first home from May 1980 to September 1982.

NURSING EDUCATION

Freed from the need to provide a basic district nursing course, the Institute is now able to concentrate its efforts and resources on post-basic district nursing education. With the changing health needs of the population, rising expectations for care, new educational concepts and new technology, such education becomes more important. The Committee of Nursing,[1] the Judge report,[2] and the Central Council's Project 2000[3] have all reiterated the need for nursing education to be seen as a continuum. As nurses have found to their cost, ignorance of new knowledge or technology is no excuse for negligence. It is small wonder, therefore, that courses, workshops and seminars with subjects as diverse as holistic care, legal and ethical aspects of district nursing, the care of the terminally ill, computers and quality assurance have all been oversubscribed. In the last five years 47 study days have been held, attended by more than 2000 nurses.

The greater potential of candidates and the more heuristic nature of the basic course now brings a demand for more highly qualified tutors and lecturers, a problem foreseen long ago when the Institute was pressing for a longer training for district nurses. In 1978, the Institute, conscious of the need to encourage a high level of community nursing input into the growing number of degree courses in nursing, and heartened by its more healthy financial position, decided to offer Chelsea College (now King's College) a grant of up to £50 000 to fund a lectureship in community nursing. The original idea was to pioneer ways of integrating community nursing into basic nurse training though this idea was not realised. This offer was accepted and the post is known as the Queen's Institute Lectureship in Community Nursing. This endowment marked a significant step forward in establishing the rightful place of district nursing in a degree-course curriculum. The first lectureship was held by Mrs Patricia Turton whose efforts ensured that the course was placed on a firm foundation and that it continued to provide district nurses with the opportunity for the further education they so needed. Now after five years the experiment has proved its worth and the University of London has assumed responsibility for funding the course.[4]

This venture was followed, in 1980 by a request from the Polytechnic of the South Bank to establish a district nurse training course that would attract students of good calibre, and who, if successful, might wish to follow up their studies with a diploma. The Institute agreed to support the course financially for three years, and in 1981 a tutor was appointed who now sits on the Council of the Institute.

Still cooperating with universities, in 1984 the Institute gave an initial grant of £11 000 to the University of Surrey to set up the Queen's Nursing Institute Resource Centre. The aim of the Centre is to promote and support the continuing education and professional development of district nurses by making available to them a central catalogue of resources. The first task has been the collection and collation of existing material and resources, and the Centre aims to produce teaching and learning aids and to mount seminars and workshops as a stimulus to research and pilot schemes.

Perhaps the most exciting of the Institute's educational ventures is the project connected with its centenary celebrations: the endowment, in conjunction with the General Nursing Council Trust and The Dowager Countess Eleanor Peel Trust, of a Chair of Community Nursing at the University of Manchester. This has largely been the inspiration of Dr Charlotte Kratz, a member of Council and before that a member of the staff of the Institute.

A chair in community nursing at a university is a far call from that experimental course offered by Miss Lees at Bloomsbury over 100 years ago; but she would have approved and so too would Miss Nightingale and William Rathbone. Over 100 years ago people fulminated against the idea of 'educating' nurses. Mr South of St Thomas's Hospital, made well-known comments[5] on 'nurses as housemaids', and today the equivalent voice may be heard, but district nurses need, and will increasingly need, a philosophical base for their work. As more people pass into longevity, living alone with disabilities beyond the scope of high technology and medical advance, so the district nurse will become a focal point of care, a counsellor and support for much of the community in its last days. It is an awesome task and it needs the best possible preparation.

The old Queen's Nurses' League was a club, and like the nurses' leagues of teaching hospitals it gave a sense of social cohesion among colleagues and many district nurses regretted its passing. Today the Queen's Institute has to find ways of giving to all district nurses that special unity it once gave to Queen's nurses. With many calls on their time professionally, both nationally and locally, and often from their own families, this is not easy. But the Institute still provides highlights in the district nurse's year when nurses can meet together socially and professionally.

THE ANNUAL MEETING

For some years now the Annual Meeting has been an open meeting at which HRH Princess Alice, Duchess of Gloucester regularly presides; it attracts a large audience to listen to lectures on subjects of interest to district nurses, such as mental handicap, nursing ethics and, more recently, discussions on the Cumberlege report and its implications for district nursing. Another feature of the Annual Meeting is the award of the Edith Bull Memorial Prize to commemorate the name of Mrs James Bull who served the Institute for thirty years, who was chairman from 1971 to 1978 and who was deeply committed to the educational activities of the Institute. Originally the award was to an outstanding fourth-year student from Chelsea College, now the net has been widened and district nurse students from any College may be nominated.

Another highlight of the district nurses' year is the presentation of the long service badges to those Queen's nurses who have completed 21 years' service in district nursing, or of the Certificate if the nurse has served fifteen years and has for some reason to leave the service. The presentation is usually made by a member of the royal family, and it is a happy occasion eagerly awaited by nurses and families alike. The ceremony goes back many years and is a link with the past.

A further way of providing district nurses with a focal meeting point, both locally and nationally, has been the foundation of the District Nursing Association. Originally set up in Scotland in 1971 under the Presidency of Lord Birsay and with much practical support from the Queen's Institute both in Edinburgh and London, it is now on a national footing and registered as a trade union, though not affiliated to the TUC. This association has close links with the Queen's Institute with its General Secretary, Jack Griffiths, on the Council, William Rathbone, Junior President, and Mrs Acland Vice-President.

PENSION SCHEMES

Throughout its existence the Queen's Institute has been much exercised by the problems of pensions and welfare provision for its nurses, who with small salaries and the hazards of the job had little chance of providing for a rainy day. Miss Loane and others may have preached the gospel of Samuel Smiles to their patients, but it was not always easy for nurses to follow their own precepts. The back pages of the *Queen's Nurses' Magazine* were full of exhortations to nurses to pay into various funds, but even when they did benefits were small. Before the war district nurses paid into life assurance schemes but inflation eroded benefits. After the coming of the National Health Service district nurses contributed to the superannuation fund, but in the early days salaries were low and benefits correspondingly meagre, and retirement for some was financially difficult.

Thanks to careful housekeeping, donations, legacies and to the great generosity of the Gardens Scheme, the Institute is able to make grants to help district nurses in need in a variety of ways.

THE NATIONAL GARDENS SCHEME

The National Gardens Scheme was started in 1927 on the imaginative suggestion of a member of the Institute's Council, Miss Elsie Wagg, to raise funds to support the welfare and benevolent function through the provision of annuities and grants. It formed part of a national memorial to Queen Alexandra, whose deep and sympathetic interest in district nursing was well known.

The Scheme grew rapidly and soon there was a nationwide network of voluntary county organisers who continually searched out new and interesting gardens to attract an increasing number of visitors, and each year generous financial help for district nurses was disbursed through the Institute itself and at a local level through county nursing associations. In 1927, 600 gardens opened raising £8 191; by 1980 1455 gardens were opening — a very large proportion on a regular annual basis — and £203 342 was raised.

By this time the Scheme had assumed a distinct horticultural ethos as well as being a charitable fund-raising organisation, and it had become inappropriate for it to remain as a department of the Institute. It was also apparent that it could, and should, widen its remit to be able to contribute to other than the Institute's benevolent funds.

In 1980, therefore, the Scheme ceased to be a subsidiary and became an independent charitable trust. Without moving its quarters from 57 Lower Belgrave Street, and with unswerving loyalty to its foundation and to the needs of District Nurses and District Nursing, it has widened its area of activity to assume the administration of Gardener's Sunday, to make generous contributions to the Macmillan Nurse Training Fund of the National Society for Cancer Relief, and to benefit many smaller charities of the garden owners' choice. The Elsie Wagg Trust supports the Institute's educational programme and the Scheme makes an annual donation through the Institute to the Nurses' Welfare Service (see p. 138).

In 1986, the year before the Institute's centenary and the Scheme's Diamond Jubilee, 2000 gardens opened to the public and over £400 000 was raised in total, of which a major proportion was contributed to the district nursing profession. The rapid enlargement and success of the Scheme since the late 1950s was due in no small part to the efforts of Rachel Crawshay, a member of the Institute's staff who became the Organising Secretary until she retired 27 years later.

So it can be easily recognised what an important part the Scheme has played in the fortunes of the Institute over the years, and how significant its support continues to be, for without this help the benevolent and welfare work would be severely curtailed.

NATION'S FUND FOR NURSES

Since 1980, the Queen's Institute has been appointed administrator of the Nation's Fund for Nurses, that source of help and succour to nurses in need since 1917. Mr Thomas Whipham, the chairman of the Fund, was appointed to the Council of the Institute, and the chairman of the Institute joined the Board of Management of the Nation's Fund. The marriage of two of the largest nursing charities, often dealing with the same needs, has led to a considerable reduction in administrative costs and allowed more money to be made available to nurses.

BENEVOLENT AND WELFARE SERVICES

In spite of the provisions of the welfare state, Beveridge's five giants are not quite dead and there are still nurses in want. With increased longevity the greatest need is with elderly nurses, some of whom may be disabled and in need of appliances. Even those with seemingly adequate pensions often cannot afford residential care when it becomes necessary, and, when all other sources are exhausted, the Queen's Institute or the Nation's Fund makes up the shortfall. However, the old are not the only nurses in need of help. Sadly, an increasing number of calls come from younger nurses who find themselves in difficulties. The occupational hazard of back injury is not new and can mean disablement and unemployment, probably at a time when family expenses are heaviest; nurses like other citizens are subject to disabling illnesses such as multiple sclerosis, and some may need permanent help.

It is not only nurses with physical disability who need help. There are now new factors in the health service that create stress. Recent changes in the management structure of the health service mean that nurses are often without nursing support in times of doubt and conflict. The primary health care team as a peer group may be supportive, but the whole team is often under stress with a heavier workload than it can tolerate. District nurses may know that they cannot deal with all the needed visits and that there is a vast area of unmet need, and this knowledge in itself creates anxiety. Public expectations rise and patients are more litigious, elderly patients are not necessarily sweet and docile, and doctors, once so wary of the encroachments of district nurses on their livelihood, now often press the district nurse to take more responsibility, for which sometimes she is not prepared. In some places the team concept is more honoured in the breach than in the observance. Most nurses are remarkably resilient and adaptable to an ever-changing situation, but some break down under the strain and need the support of a welfare service, and the personal touch of one of the Institute's professional advisers.

In a property-owning democracy district nurses like other citizens have mortgages and fuel bills, and when illness or redundancy come to them or their family the commitments continue. The Queen's nurse of yesteryear was invariably single, she often lived in a rented cottage owned and provided by her Association, she may have had paid help and when ill, if lucky, she was sent to Bryn-y-Menai and usually supported until she returned. In many ways life was simpler; charity it may have been, but the world we have lost was not without its compensations. Now, even if the economic position of the district nurse improves, the pressures on the service are likely to be such, together with the rising 'conspicuous consumption', that there will be a continuing need for a source of help for district and other nurses in times of need.

THE NURSES' WELFARE SERVICE

Since 1976 the Institute has been associated with the Nurses' Welfare Service. This had been set up in 1972 to assist any nurse who became involved in, or was at risk of becoming involved in, the disciplinary procedures of the General Nursing Council. From 1976 to 1979 the Service was housed, administered and largely funded by the Institute, but by 1980 the increased workload of the Service required fresh arrangements to be made for its expanding future. It was therefore decided that an independent trust should be established with responsibility for the Service and that it should move to premises owned by and near to the GNC. Although the Institute is no longer directly connected with the Service, it still makes a substantial contribution to its work each year with money allocated by the National Gardens Scheme.

ENCOURAGING UNITY

The Institute's other important role today is to encourage unity in the nursing profession and particularly in the primary care team. The first district nurses 100 years ago were 'all purpose health workers', but at the beginning of this century they began to lose some of their functions to other professions, a difficulty made worse by the fact that the other groups were accountable to different employers and there was often little communication between workers dealing with the same clients. Inevitably there were gaps, overlaps and demarcation disputes which the Registration Act of 1919 did nothing to resolve. Nothing was done to coordinate or unify post-basic trainings which grew like the many-headed hydra. It took 60 years to slay the monster, and Hercules finally arrived in the form of the Central Council when it assumed responsibility for no less than nine different training bodies and councils. The nursing profession has been factious and fissiparous, but with the new emphasis on the holistic approach it is important to put faction aside.

The Queen's Institute has long been aware of the need for district nurses, health visitors and school nurses to work amicably together and for unity in the primary care team. We cannot complain about the lack of cooperation from the doctors when the nursing team itself is at odds. For this reason the Institute welcomed government agreement for a review of community nursing to be carried out in England. The review team, to which the Institute gave evidence, was chaired by Mrs Julia Cumberlege and their report was issued in 1986.[8]

With minor reservations the Institute has welcomed the report which reinforces the view that the interests of patients and families are best served when district nurses, health visitors and general practitioners work together in effective primary health care teams. To further this development the report recommends that the UKCC and English National Board should: 'introduce a common training course for all first-level nurses wishing to work outside hospital in what are now the fields of health visiting, district nursing and school nursing'.[8] After this there should be an option to take specialist modules which would lead to the nurse's name being placed on the register and all parts would have equal value.

The Institute endorses these recommendations for they would go a long way towards bringing unity to the profession and a greater understanding between colleagues. If doctors accept the underlying philosophy they could be relieved of some of their work and the public would get a better service. It is appropriate that the Queen's Institute should celebrate its centenary with the hope that the primary health services should become paramount and the nursing team should be unified. Miss Lees designed that core curriculum 100 years ago, and all it needs is to be updated to meet the needs of the year 2000.

In 1860 a Mrs Mary Robinson, at the behest of Mr William Rathbone, went out into the slums of Liverpool to try and bring nursing care to the sick poor and returned in tears, overwhelmed by the misery she saw. Today, to celebrate its centenary, the Institute arranged for a Mrs Edna Robinson from Manchester to spend a month with the Visiting Nurse Association in Boston, United States seeing aspects of community care there, and in 1987 the Institute will be receiving a nurse from Boston for a four-week return visit. Thus the Institute keeps up its long tradition of furthering the cause of district nursing beyond these shores.

This history is a testament to the 100 years of achievement of the Queen's Nursing Institute, from its inception as the Queen Victoria's Jubilee Institute for Nurses in the three rooms in that neo-Gothic establishment in Regent's Park, through many vicissitudes, to its present home in Belgravia. It is the story of the struggle to establish something that was revolutionary. A district nursing service that was secular, independent of class and creed, and totally non-sectarian, where hospital-trained nurses were accepted on grounds of aptitude and general education, and who were specifically trained as health missionaries to meet the needs of the poor in their own homes. The training aimed at a standard of excellence with 'a higher and better training than that provided by hospital training'. The original Queen's nurses were a small group, but they soon became a standard for emulation. This standard did eventually spread through the whole land as Miss Nightingale told Mr Rathbone it would, largely due to the efforts and vigilance of the Institute, its Council, its long history of outstanding officers and to those often unsung superintendents who turned 'nurses' into 'Queen's nurses'.

NOTES

1. *The Report of the Committee on Nursing*, HMSO, London, Cmnd 5115, 1970.

2. *Education of Nurses: A new Dispensation* (Judge report), RCN, London, 1985.

3. *Project 2000*, UKCC, London, 1986.

4. Queen's Nursing Institute Annual Reports, 1978–84.

5. Woodham-Smith, C. *Florence Nightingale*, Constable, London, 1960, p. 345.

6. The District Nursing Association (UK). Aims of the Association.

7. Report of the National Gardens Scheme Annual Meeting, November, 1986.

8. *Neighbourhood Nursing — A Focus for Care* (Cumberlege report) HMSO, London, 1986.

12

Epilogue

A hundred years ago the early Queen's nurses battled to put the rooms of the sick poor in nursing order. Nurses writing home told of heart-breaking stories of little children dying from fever lying in indescribable Dickensian squalor, and of drunken fathers resisting their entry as they arrived in the fog on the doorstep.[1] Miss Lees' case books are full of stories of 'neglect, dirt and stench that bred fever'. With the aid of carbolic, soap and water, threats to recalcitrant landlords and references to charities, the main mission was to bring better sanitation, feeding, fresh air and hope to the poor. The poor often could not afford a doctor; and more often, if they could the doctor could do little, the cause of the sickness lay in the environment and the social conditions of the poor. Miss Nightingale asked the question 'Is the district nurse in any sense a doctor?' not because she wanted nurses to usurp doctors but because she questioned the main purpose of medicine. Doctors, in her opinion, did not understand the sanitary mission and they failed to tackle the real causes of ill-health.

In the intervening years medicine became more scientific. Thanks to the validation of the germ theory, eventually most bacterial disease could be prevented or cured. The standard of living improved, the water closet and a clean water supply put an end to water-borne diseases. Hospitals began to lose their terrors. There were hospitals for fevers, hospitals for children and that ubiquitous manifestation of local pride, the cottage hospital; there was less need for district nurses to prepare for operations on the kitchen table. Meantime health care in the community and the sanitary mission split into factions, different workers took over tasks that had once been performed by the district nurse, and doctors competed for patients. The story of district nursing over the first 87 years of the century has been that of adapting to change, and the story of the Institute has been that of finding resources to prepare nurses to meet the change.

Now the wheel has come full circle. The realisation that hospitals create dependency, that they cost twice as much as an expensive hotel and that they cannot be relied on 'to do the patient no harm' means that they are used as little as possible and that the patient's stay is short. The district nurse may not have to assist with operations in the kitchen but now she does have post-operative care. People can now afford a doctor, but, like Miss Lees' patients, is it always a doctor they need? Many people have suggested, and it is now enshrined in the Cumberlege report, that the burden of general practice might be relieved if patients had a choice of seeing either the doctor or the nurse. Tomorrow's patients may make a conscious choice to consult a nurse.

Today, instead of sick children, the district nurse's greatest caseload comes from the elderly, and as people live longer they will have more episodes of ill-health, and the need for community care is rising faster than the resources to meet it. Having cured what can be cured and prevented what society will allow to be prevented, what is left is care, and much of the burden of care will fall upon the district nurse and the family or the neighbours who must be supported and instructed, a point today's nurses have in common with their predecessors.

There are, of course, many striking differences between 1887 and 1987. For one thing we have exchanged the diseases of scarcity for those of affluence. Secondly, in 1887 doctors and nurses could do little about the main scourges of the day; today the district nurse has in her armoury a range of powerful prescribed drugs and high technology, one reason why errors on the part of the nurse are now so much more dangerous — her capacity for harm through a mistake is infinitely greater. Third, and perhaps most important, is the fact that the early Queen's nurses came almost exclusively to the poor sick; today the district nurse is the prescriber and giver of care to all walks of society, a development that would have pleased Sir Henry Ponsonby who wanted Queen's nurses for the Palace. The brigadier coping with his Parkinson's disease and his bereavement is as much in need of the district nurse as the manual worker after his stroke, but this diversity calls for adaptability with social and communication skills of a high order, skills that are not necessarily always inculcated in the basic training.[2]

And yet much remains the same, *plus ça change — plus c'est la même chose*. There is no longer the depressing squalor of the nineteenth-century slums, but in areas of high unemployment and in the inner cities, housing conditions are often appalling and there is still much homelessness. High-rise flats, that Mecca for vandals, have in some areas replaced the old courts in squalor, and tenants are afraid to go out. The early district nurses were much concerned with the effects of ophthalmia neonatorum and other effects of venereal disease. These have largely disappeared, but now the problem of AIDS rears its head and no one knows how large it may loom in the future. Today we are not concerned with 'little blossoms gathered to the angels', but there needs to be constant vigilance about child abuse, and 100 years after Dickens horrified his readers with tales of child cruelty children are still battered to death. The early district nurses sometimes coped with drunken abuse but generally their uniform protected them today the uniform may attract violence because it is thought that nurses carry drugs. With the return of many mentally handicapped people to the community the district nurse is back to the position of her predecessors.

In spite of the advances of medicine, new technology, the changed social conditions and the concept of a primary health care team, the factors that unite district nurses with their past are greater than those that divide. The district nurse is still the guest in the patient's home and can only give service if she is accepted. Only by looking back along the road from which they have come can district nurses and the Queen's Institute take their bearings and look for a signpost to the road along which they must now travel.

NOTES

1. GLRO HI/ST/NTS/Y16.1, The Cadbury Letters, 1877–79.
2. Stockwell, F., *The Unpopular Patient*, RCN, London, 1973.

Select Bibliography

PRIMARY SOURCES

Held at the Queen's Nursing Institute   Institute of Nursing Sisters (fd.1840)
Records of Nurses', Queen's (Commemoration) Fund, Queen Mary's Committee, Visible Memorial to Queen Alexandra, Records of Affiliation of Local Associations, Records of Federations and Affiliated Associations, Queen's Nurses' Association, Association of Queen's Superintendents, Miscellaneous volumes.
Files: Historic — largely collected for Mary Stocks' book
      Archives — General   QNI
Held at the British Library Department of Manuscripts   BL
The Nightingale collection notably the Nightingale/Rathbone correspondence.
Held at the Public Record Office, Kew   PRO
Inspectors' reports of the Queen's Institute of District Nursing 1897–1944. Filed by area.
Held at the Greater London Record Office   GLRO
The Nightingale collection, Nightingale Fund Council records, the Bonham Carter collection.
Held at the Brown Picton and Hornby Libraries Liverpool
Records relating to the Liverpool District Nursing Association and the Rathbone Staff College. Some Nightingale/Rathbone correspondence (mostly duplicates of the BL).

JOURNALS

Nursing Notes   selected copies
Nursing Mirror   selected copies
Nursing Times   selected copies
Queen's Nurses' Magazine 1904–58
District Nursing Journal 1958–77
The Lancet and *British Medical Journal*   selected copies

SELECT REPORTS

The Report of the Lancet Commission 1932
(Chairman: The Earl of Crawford and Balcarres) *The Lancet*
Interdepartmental Committee on Nursing Services
(Chairman: The Rt Hon. The Earl of Athlone) 1939   HMSO
Working Party on the Recruitment and Training of Nurses
(Chairman: Sir Robert Wood) Majority Report 1947   HMSO
Working Party on Training of District Nurses
(Chairman: R. Ingall) 1955   HMSO

145

An Enquiry into Health Visiting
(Chairman: Sir Wilson Jameson) 1956   HMSO
Future Scope of General Practice
(Chairman: Dr A. Gillie) 1963
Management Structure in the Local Health Authority Nursing Services
(Chairman: E. Mayston) 1969   DHSS
The Organisation of Group Practice
(Chairman: Dr R. Harvard Davies) 1971   HMSO
The Committee on Nursing
(Chairman: Professor Asa Briggs) 1972   HMSO
Working Party Report of the Panel of Assessors
Education and Training of District Nurses 1976
Project 2000
(Chairman: Dr C. Davies) 1986   UKCC
Neighbourhood Nursing — A Focus for Care
(Chairman: Mrs Julia Cumberlege) 1986   HMSO

LEAFLETS AND BOOKLETS

Liverpool Queen Victoria Nursing Association (Founded 1898) London,
Hudson and Keans.   UD
On Trained Nursing for the Sick Poor (Introduction: F. Nightingale) (1881)
London, Spottiswoode and Co.
On Trained Nursing for the Sick Poor in *The Times* (April 1876) (Plea for
support for the Metropolitan Nursing Association)   BL
Organisation of Nursing — An Account of Liverpool Nursing (Introduction:
F. Nightingale) UD Picton Library
Leading Article reprinted from *The Times* (23 March 1908)
District Nursing in Towns (1884) Mary Minet, London, Spottiswoode and Co.
District Nursing in the Homes of the Poor (1896) L. Twining
The Story of the Queen's Nurses in Scotland (?1920) Edinburgh, Lindsay
and Co.
District Nursing on a Provident Basis (1910) Amy Hughes, London, Spottis-
woode and Co.
Suggestions as to the Provident Method of Support of District Nursing
(UD?1920s), Queen's Institute of District Nursing
Queen Victoria's Jubilee Institute for Nurses (1913) London, Lowe Bros.
A Morning with a Queen's Nurse by a Looker-on (UD) London, Lowe Bros.
The Queen's Nurses during the Second World War (1945) Mercy Wilmshurst,
London, Letchworth
Educational Services (1976)   Queen's Nursing Institute
*Report and Proceedings of the Jubilee Congress on District Nursing in Liver-
pool*, Marples & Co. (1909)

BOOKS

Abel-Smith B. (1960) *A History of the Nursing Profession*. London,
  Heinemann.

Baly M.E. (1986) *Florence Nightingale and the Nursing Legacy*. London, Croom Helm.

Baly M.E., Clark J., Robottom D. and Chapple M. (1981) *A New Approach to District Nursing*. London, Heinemann.

Briggs A. (1975) *Victorian People*. Harmondsworth, Pelican.

Craven, Dacre F. (1890) *A Guide to District Nursing and Home Nursing*. London, Macmillan.

Cresswell, F. (1883) *A Memoir of Elizabeth Fry*. London, J. Nisbett.

Davies C. ed. (1980) *Rewriting Nursing History*. London, Croom Helm.

Donnison J. (1977) *Midwives and Medical Men*. London, Macmillan.

Handbook for District Nurses (1924) Various authors. London, Faber and Faber.

Hardy G. (1981) *William Rathbone and the Early History of District Nursing*. Ormskirk, G.W. and A. Hesketh.

Hurry J.B. (1898) *District Nursing on a Provident Basis*. London, Scientific Press.

Jamison C. (1952) *The History of the Royal Hospital of St Katherine's*. London, Oxford University Press.

Lamb A. (1977) *Primary Health Nursing*. London, Baillière Tindall.

Loane M. (1906) *From Their Point of View*. London, Edward Arnold.

—— (1907) *The Next Street But One*. London, Edward Arnold.

—— (1909) *The Queen's Poor*. London, Edward Arnold.

Malleson H. (1926) *The Life of Elizabeth Malleson*. 1828–1916, privately printed.

Merry E.J. and Irven I.D. (1948) *District Nursing*. London, Baillière Tindall and Cox.

Platt E. (1939) *The Story of the Ranyard Mission*. London, Hodder and Stoughton.

Rathbone E. (1904) *William Rathbone — A Memoir*. London, Macmillan.

Rathbone W. (1890) *The History and Progress of District Nursing* (dedicated to Her Majesty Queen Victoria), London, Macmillan.

—— (1967) *The Story of a Successful Experiment*. London, Macmillan.

—— (1900) *A Short History of District Nursing in Liverpool*. Liverpool, Marples and Co.

Rose J. (1980) *Elizabeth Fry*. London, Macmillan.

Simey M.B. (1951) *Charitable Efforts in Liverpool in the Nineteenth Century*. Liverpool University.

Smith F. (1982) *Florence Nightingale — Reputation and Power*. London, Croom Helm.

Stocks M. (1960) *A Hundred Years of District Nursing*. London, Allen and Unwin.

White R. (1985) *The Effects of the NHS on the Nursing Profession*. London, King Edward's Hospital Fund.

Woodham-Smith C. (1950) *Florence Nightingale*. London, Constable.

Appendix

A Hundred Years of District Nursing

1874 Metropolitan and National Nursing Association founded with Miss Lees as Superintendent on the advice of Mr William Rathbone and Miss Nightingale.

1887 Queen Victoria's Golden Jubilee; £70 000 collected for the Women's Jubilee Offering.

1888 The Rural District Nursing Association founded.

1889 The Queen Victoria's Jubilee Institute for Nurses granted a Royal Charter.

1897 Queen Victoria's Diamond Jubilee; 539 Queen's nurses on the Roll. Commemoration Fund produces £68 000.

1901 Death of Queen Victoria.

1902 Village nurse midwife training organised at Plaistow, East London.

1904 The *Queen's Nurses' Magazine* first published.
The Queen Victoria's Jubilee Institute severs its connection with St Katherine's. New headquarters at 120 Victoria Street.

1909 The Liverpool Jubilee Congress on District Nursing.
The Report of the Poor Law Commission.

1912 The Highlands and Islands medical service in Scotland.

1914 Start of the First World War — Queen's nurses join the armed services.

1916 The College of Nursing founded.

1918 Maternity and Child Welfare Act. Local authorities required to provide nurses for infectious diseases.

1919 Nurses Registration Act. Queen's nurses asked to register.

1925 Queen Victoria's Jubilee Institute becomes the Queen's Institute of District Nursing.

1926 Death of Queen Alexandra — The Memorial Fund launched.

1927 The Gardens Scheme inaugurated by Miss E. Wragg.

1928 Supplementary Charter issued to the Queen's Institute of District Nursing.

1933 The Queen's Institute moves its headquarters to 57 Lower Belgrave Street, London.
LCC report on District Nursing in London.

1936 The Midwives Act.

1939 The Athlone Report (suggests the introduction of the assistant nurse).

Outbreak of the Second World War.

1943 The Rushcliffe Committee — Queen's nurses get new salaries.

1947 The Queen's Institute offers training to male nurses.

1948 The National Health Service inaugurated. Local health authorities become responsible for supplying a 'home nursing service'.

1953 Working Party on district nurse training under the chairmanship of Sir Frederick Armer.

1955 Working Party on the training of district nurses under R. Ingall. Formation of the panel of assessors and the award of a National Certificate of District Nursing.

1956 The Jameson Report on health visiting.

1959 The revision of the General Nursing Council's syllabus, student nurses to have five days' community observation.

1960 The William Rathbone Staff College opened.

1967 The Queen's Institute of District Nursing withdraws from training responsibilities.

The Mayston Report: *Management Structure in the Local Authority Nursing Service.* Introduction of the grade of nursing officer for district nursing sisters with wide experience.

1970 Arrangements for extending district training to state enrolled nurses.

1972 *The Committee on Nursing* (Briggs) plans for the training and education of nurses in Higher Education.

Circular 25/72 revises syllabus of training for the state registered nurse in district training.

1973 National Health Service Reorganisation Act. District nursing sisters employed by area health authorities.

1974 Panel of assessors for district nurse training issues *Handbook for Training*; education centres set up.

1975 The William Rathbone Staff College closed.

1976 Working Party report of the panel of assessors on Education and Training of District Nurses. Proposed that outline syllabus replace the existing syllabus (Carr).

The Queen's Nursing Institute assumes responsibility for the administration and funding of the Nurses' Welfare Service.

Report on the *Future of Child Health Services* (Court).

1979 The Queen's Nursing Institute Lectureship in Community

Nursing established at Chelsea College, University of London.

Nurses, Midwives and Health Visitors Act.

1980 The new curriculum on district nurse training issued.

The National Gardens Scheme becomes an independent charitable trust.

1981 New curriculum comes into force.

First award of the Edith Bull Memorial Prize to a district nurse student for 'excellent patient care and high academic achievement'.

The Queen's Nursing Institute accepts responsibility for the administration of the Nation's Fund for Nurses and its associated charities.

Institute funding of a District Nurse Tutor at the Polytechnic of the South Bank, London.

1981–82 Arrangements for restructuring the National Health Service into District Health Authorities under the provisions of the Health Services Act (1980).

1983 The Griffiths Reorganisation. The concept of general managers introduced.

The United Kingdom Central Council for Nursing, Midwifery and Health Visiting and the four National Boards established. The Council and Boards replaced the nine statutory and training bodies that had previously been responsible for nursing education.

1985 *The Education of Nurses — A New Dispensation* (Judge Report) issued by the Royal College of Nursing.

1986 *Project 2000* issued by the United Kingdom Central Council.

Neighbourhood Nursing — A Focus for Care, the report of the Cumberlege Committee sets forth proposals for the future of the primary health care nursing team.

1987 The Queen's Nursing Institute celebrates its centenary.

Queen's Nursing Institute Chair of Community Nursing established at Manchester University.

Index